The Efficacy and Safety of M

Louisa Maja Hauenstein

The Efficacy and Safety of Misoprostol in Obstetrics

An overview of the last twenty years of use

Natural Sciences Series

Impressum / Imprint
Bibliografische Information der Deutschen Nationalbibliothek: Die Deutsche Nationalbibliothek verzeichnet diese Publikation in der Deutschen Nationalbibliografie; detaillierte bibliografische Daten sind im Internet über http://dnb.d-nb.de abrufbar.
Alle in diesem Buch genannten Marken und Produktnamen unterliegen warenzeichen-, marken- oder patentrechtlichem Schutz bzw. sind Warenzeichen oder eingetragene Warenzeichen der jeweiligen Inhaber. Die Wiedergabe von Marken, Produktnamen, Gebrauchsnamen, Handelsnamen, Warenbezeichnungen u.s.w. in diesem Werk berechtigt auch ohne besondere Kennzeichnung nicht zu der Annahme, dass solche Namen im Sinne der Warenzeichen- und Markenschutzgesetzgebung als frei zu betrachten wären und daher von jedermann benutzt werden dürften.

Bibliographic information published by the Deutsche Nationalbibliothek: The Deutsche Nationalbibliothek lists this publication in the Deutsche Nationalbibliografie; detailed bibliographic data are available in the Internet at http://dnb.d-nb.de.
Any brand names and product names mentioned in this book are subject to trademark, brand or patent protection and are trademarks or registered trademarks of their respective holders. The use of brand names, product names, common names, trade names, product descriptions etc. even without a particular marking in this works is in no way to be construed to mean that such names may be regarded as unrestricted in respect of trademark and brand protection legislation and could thus be used by anyone.

Coverbild / Cover image: www.ingimage.com

Verlag / Publisher:
AV Akademikerverlag
ist ein Imprint der / is a trademark of
OmniScriptum GmbH & Co. KG
Heinrich-Böcking-Str. 6-8, 66121 Saarbrücken, Deutschland / Germany
Email: info@akademikerverlag.de

Herstellung: siehe letzte Seite /
Printed at: see last page
ISBN: 978-3-639-49955-1

Copyright © 2014 OmniScriptum GmbH & Co. KG
Alle Rechte vorbehalten. / All rights reserved. Saarbrücken 2014

Table of Content

1. Abstract 6
2. Introduction 8
   2.1 Misoprostol in General 8
      2.1.1 Characteristics 8
      2.1.2 Pharmacokinetics 9
   2.2 Misoprostol in Pregnancy 10
      2.2.1 Mechanism of Action 10
      2.2.2 Indications 10
      2.2.3 Adverse Drug Reactions (ADR) 13
   2.3 Off-label Use 14
      2.3.1 Off-label Use in General 14
      2.3.2 Off-label Use in Pregnancy 15
   2.4 Aim of this Study 16
3. Material and Methods 17
   3.1 Search Strategy in PubMed Database 17
   3.2 Selection of Studies 18
      3.2.1 Study Population 18
      3.2.2 Study Designs 19
      3.2.3 Language 21
      3.2.4 Excluded Studies 21
   3.3 Description and Analysis of the Included Studies 21

    3.3.1 Database 21

    3.3.2 Analysed Aspects 27

    3.3.3 Statistical Methods 28

4. Results 29

  4.1 Overview 29

    4.1.1 Studies 29

    4.1.2 Women 32

  4.2 Maternal Adverse Drug Reactions (ADR) 34

    4.2.1 Overview 34

    4.2.2 Maternal ADR by Trimester of Pregnancy 35

    4.2.3 Maternal ADR by Indication 39

    4.2.4 Maternal ADR by different Modes of Application of Misoprostol 42

    4.2.5 Maternal ADR by different Doses 46

    4.2.6 Maternal ADR with Misoprostol alone vs. in Combination with Oxytocin 47

    4.2.7 Maternal ADR by Evaluation of RCTs only 51

  4.3 Maternal Serious Adverse (Drug) Reactions (SAR) 52

  4.4 Delivery 61

    4.4.1 Overview 61

    4.4.2 Delivery Outcome by Trimester of Pregnancy 62

    4.4.3 Delivery Outcome by Indications 65

    4.4.4 Delivery Outcome by different Modes of Application of Misoprostol 67

4.4.5 Delivery Outcome by different Doses ... 69

4.4.6 Delivery Outcome with Misoprostol alone vs. in Combination with Oxytocin ... 71

4.5 Neonatal Outcome ... 75

4.5.1 Overview ... 75

4.5.2 Neonatal ADR by different Modes of Application of Misoprostol ... 76

4.5.3 Neonatal ADR by different Doses ... 77

4.6 Performed Meta-analyses of Maternal Adverse Drug Reactions and Delivery ... 79

4.6.1 GIT Disturbances ... 79

4.6.2 Fever and Shivering ... 84

4.6.3 Hyperstimulation Syndrome (Uterine Contraction Abnormalities with Foetal Heart-Rate Changes) ... 89

4.6.4 Caesarean Section (CS) ... 92

5. Discussion ... 96

5.1 Maternal Adverse Drug Reactions (ADR) ... 96

5.2 Delivery ... 101

5.3 Neonatal Outcome ... 102

5.4 Strengths and Weaknesses of this Study ... 103

5.5 Appraisal of the off-label Use by the Legal Authority (Swissmedic) ... 105

6. References ... 109

6.1 Analysed Studies ... 109

6.2 References ... 170

7. Abbreviations 173

8. Appendix 175

Acknowledgements

I would like to give special thanks to:

The University Hospital of Zurich, Department of Obstetrics, for giving me the opportunity to realise this work.

Prof. Dr. Ursula von Mandach, Department of Obstetrics and Gynecology University of Zurich, for her broad and unfailing support and her constant belief in my work.

Prof. Dr. Burkhard Seifert, Department of Biostatistics Zurich, for an enormous amount of time and his most patient support.

Dr. Friederike Grimm, Dr. med. Hans Stötter, and Dr. Urs Kopp, Swissmedic, for their interest in our project and their readiness to give me detailed information on the process of transferring a drug from off-label to licensed use.

Corina von Arx and Yvonne Eisenegger for helping me with the transcription of the meeting with the experts of Swissmedic.

Marco Knaus for helping me organise and format the text.

And finally, my family and friends for their constant support and encouragement.

1. Abstract

Background

Misoprostol (Cytotec ®) is a prostaglandin analogue which was developed for the prevention and treatment of gastroduodenal ulcers. Due to its properties of inducing ripening of the cervix and contractions of the pregnant uterus, it has also been found to be a very useful drug for several important indications in obstetrics. Although it is frequently used in many countries of the world, including Switzerland, it is still not licensed for these indications and therefore in off-label use.

In the last twenty years, profound research has been conducted, leaving a considerable number of studies and data describing the use of misoprostol in obstetrics. Nevertheless, its use is still being discussed, as there are also repeated reports on serious adverse drug reactions, such as uterine rupture and maternal death, following the use of misoprostol in pregnant women. Worldwide, there is great discrepancy in the trust in its efficacy and safety. In Switzerland, but also in many developing countries, it is one of the most important and frequently used drugs in obstetrics, whereas in other countries, such as Germany or Italy, it has already been completely withdrawn from sale.

Material and Methods

By pooling and evaluating data from studies investigating the use of misoprostol in its three main obstetrical indications (namely cervical ripening and labour induction, abortion induction, as well as the prevention and treatment of postpartum haemorrhage), published in the online database PubMed from 1987 until 2011, an overview of the available information on the efficacy and safety of misoprostol in obstetrics was provided. Evaluated aspects include administrative information on the analysed studies, study population, description of the use of misoprostol, the association between misoprostol and adverse drug reactions (ADR) in mother and child, as well as outcome of birth.

Results

Overall, the occurrence of the most frequently observed maternal ADR, namely gastrointestinal ADR (in up to 53.4%) and fever and shivering (in up to 42.7%), was shown to be dependent on the dose as well as on the mode of application of misoprostol. Gastrointestinal ADR were significantly more common after oral (RR random = 1.9, CI 95%: 1.17-3.09) and after sublingual (RR random = 1.24, CI 95%: 1.02-1.51) than after vaginal application. Fever and shivering occurred significantly more frequently after a higher-dose regimen of vaginal misoprostol (RR random 1.16, CI 95%: 1.07-1.25). Hyperstimulation syndrome also occurred more frequently after higher doses (RR random = 0.61, CI 95%: 0.31-1.21) and after vaginal misoprostol when compared to PGE2 (RR random = 1.31, CI 95%: 0.94-1.83), although these results were not statistically significant. The risk of caesarean section was significantly decreased, when oral misoprostol was compared to placebo (RR random = 0.61, CI 95%: 0.42-0.89) and to PGE2 (RR random = 0.84, CI 95%: 0.74-0.96). In the overall population of 126'477 analysed women treated with misoprostol, there were 67 cases of uterine rupture and 29 cases of maternal death. The occurrence of neonatal ADR could not been clearly related to the dose and mode of application of misoprostol.

Conclusion

Misoprostol plays an important role in obstetrics in Switzerland and many other countries of the world. Its efficacy and safety are similar or better compared to other drugs used for the described indications. However, different (serious) ADR are known to occur, dependent on the mode of application and dose of misoprostol. It is therefore important to know these ADR, in order to prevent them and to be able to react in time, should they occur. Following these preventive measures, the off-label use of misoprostol can be configured more safely.

2. Introduction

2.1 Misoprostol in General

Molecular formula of misoprostol [1]

2.1.1 Characteristics

- IUPAC: methyl 7-((1R, 2R, 3R)-3-hydroxy-2-((S.E)-4-hydroxy-4-methyloct-1-enyl)-5-oxocyclopentyl)-heptanoate
- Chemical formula: $C_2H_{38}O_5$
- Molecular weight: 383.5 g/mol
- Misoprostol was developed by Searle in 1973 and was introduced to the market in 1985 under the brand name of Cytotec ® [2].

Misoprostol is a synthetic analogue of prostaglandin E1. It was developed for the treatment of peptic ulcers and the prevention and treatment of gastric and duodenal ulcers resulting from chronic use of non-steroidal antiiflammatory drugs (NSAIDs), due to its inhibition of gastric acid and pepsin secretion and various mucosa-protective properties. Its use for this indication is contraindicated for pregnant women, because it may cause uterine contractions and is associated with abortion, premature birth of the child, intrauterine foetal death, and birth defects [3].

Misoprostol has several advantages over other prostaglandins used in different indications:

- It has no effect on the blood vessels or the bronchi.
- It is very stable, therefore does not require refrigeration and can be stored at room temperature for many years.
- It can be administered by different routes (e.g. oral, vaginal, sublingual, or rectal).
- Since misoprostol is licensed for the prevention and treatment of peptic ulcers, it is widely used and easily available also in many developing countries.
- It is much less expensive than other prostaglandin analogues [2, 4, 5, 6].

2.1.2 Pharmacokinetics

After absorption, the drug undergoes a first-pass metabolism in the liver and is deesterificated to free misoprostol acid, which is the principal and active metabolite of the drug. Independent of its dose, a high proportion of the drug (<90%) is bound to plasma proteins. 75% of the drug are eliminated as an inactive polar metabolite in the urine. The remaining 15% are egested by the intestinal route [3, 5].

After **oral** administration, the drug is rapidly and almost completely absorbed by the gastrointestinal tract [5]. The plasma concentration reaches a peak after 27.5 ± 14.8 min (tmax). The terminal elimination half-life is 20-40 min [4].

After **vaginal** application, the effects occur slower than after oral application. The peak of plasma concentration is reached after 72.0 ± 34.5 min and sinks with a half-life time of 4 h [3]. The area under the plasma-concentration-versus-time curve (AUC) has been found to be significantly higher after vaginal than after oral administration [5].

After **rectal** application, the pharmacokinetics are similar to those after vaginal application, and a peak in concentration can be observed after 45-120 min. The concentration sinks slowly. The maximum plasma concentrations are lower after rectal application than after vaginal application [4].

After **sublingual** application, the pharmacokinetics are similar to those after oral application, with a tmax after 26.0 ± 11.5 min [3]. Of all application modes, sublingual application has the shortest tmax, reaches the highest peak concentration, and has the highest bioavailability [7].

2.2 Misoprostol in Pregnancy

2.2.1 Mechanism of Action

In the pregnant uterus, misoprostol shows a selective binding to the three subtypes of prostaglandin E receptors, with an affinity of PGE-R3 > PGE-R2 > PGE-R1. The binding of misoprostol to these receptors causes contractions of the uterine smooth muscle and induces ripening of the cervix. For this reason, misoprostol can also be used for different obstetrical indications [2], [4].

2.2.2 Indications

There are three major indications for misoprostol in obstetrics:

- Induction of cervical ripening and labour induction at term
- Abortion induction
- Prevention and treatment of PPH

Cervical Ripening and Labour Induction
During pregnancy and labour, as well as in the postpartum period, there is an intensive physiological reorganisation of the cervix. Unlike the

corpus of the uterus, which mainly contains smooth muscle cells, the cervical tissue consists principally of connective tissue. The cervix is therefore usually rather inelastic, but during labour, it has to dilate rapidly, and its walls become very thin, soft and vulnerable. These enormous changes occur not only passively through the pressure of labour, but are the consequence of a constant, active biochemical process of maturation during late pregnancy. Under the influence of different humoral factors (namely oestrogen, progesterone, nitric oxide, and also prostaglandins), water is retained within the cervical tissue, and collagen fibres are reorganised and partially digested by proteases. This leads to a softening and increased flexibility of the tissue, so that, finally, the mechanical influence of the uterine contractions results in dilatation of the cervix and opening of the cervical os [8].

The spontaneous onset of labour at term is induced by various placental and foetal hormones, such as oestrogen and progesterone, but also prostaglandins E2 and F2. During labour, the release of oxytocin from the maternal posterior pituitary is increased. Simultaneously, the myometrium expresses an augmented number of oxytocin receptors, which further stimulates the ongoing and increasing action of labour [9].

Besides cervical ripening, misoprostol is also used prior to surgical termination of pregnancy in the first and second trimester. Several studies have shown that softening of the cervix decreases in the duration of the surgical procedure. This might be especially important in the case of abortion at an increased gestational age, where mechanical dilatation takes longer and is more difficult [10].

Abortion Induction

Due to its labour-inducing properties, misoprostol can also be used as an abortifacient. It is used for induction of abortion in the first (0-12 weeks) and the second (13-24 weeks) trimester of pregnancy for voluntary interruption of pregnancy or after intrauterine foetal death. The application of misoprostol for abortion induction is only licensed when combined with mifepristone (Mifegyne ®), a progesterone-receptor antagonist [4].

Misoprostol is further used for uterine evacuation after incomplete and missed abortion. For these indications, misoprostol is listed under the „essential drugs" by the WHO [11].

Prevention and Treatment of Postpartum Haemorrhage (PPH)

Postpartum haemorrhage (PPH) is still one of the major factors influencing maternal morbidity and mortality in puerperium, both in developed and developing countries [12]. PPH is defined as a blood loss greater than 500 ml [13]. The most common cause of PPH is uterine atony [13].

An active management of the third stage of labour is therefore very important and commonly practised. Standard management includes early cord clamping, uterine massage, placental delivery by controlled cord traction, and routine administration of an oxytocic drug [13]. This may be oxytocin (which is the standard drug in many hospitals), but also misoprostol, which significantly reduces the incidence of PPH when administered routinely after childbirth compared with placebo [14].

Since PPH is a life-threatening complication, immediate treatment is absolutely necessary. There are several treatment options, including medical methods with uterotonics (such as ergometrine, oxytocin, or prostaglandins), surgical tying off or blocking of the uterine artery, or the administration of haemostatic drugs [15]. For the treatment of PPH, misoprostol has been tried in several studies, but it is still under assessment and has not yet proved to have advantages over other methods [16].

As illustrated above, misoprostol plays a very important role and is widely used in obstetrics. Nevertheless, the current patent holder Pfizer has never applied to get a licence for Cytotec ® for any of the mentioned obstetrical indications. In most countries, also in Switzerland, misoprostol is therefore used as an off-label drug. Only France, Egypt, Brazil, and Taiwan have licensed dedicated products for gynaecological and obstetrical use [2,4].

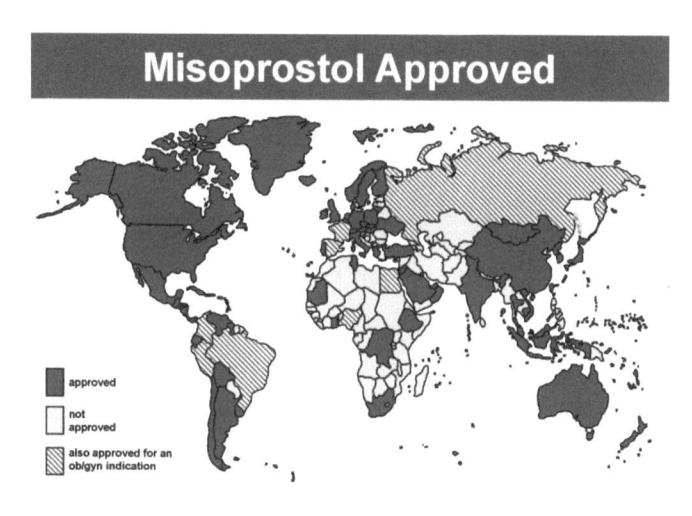

Worldwide approval of misoprostol [17].

2.2.3 Adverse Drug Reactions (ADR)

Common ADR

The most commonly observed adverse drug reactions (ADR) of misoprostol are nausea, vomiting, diarrhoea, abdominal pain, chills, shivering and fever. They are all dose-dependent [18].

ADR in Pregnancy, Birth and the Puerperium

In pregnant women, misoprostol may cause abnormal uterine contractions (tachysystolia, hypersystolia, and hyperstimulation), uterine bleeding, perforation or rupture of the uterus, retention of the placenta, amniotic fluid embolism, incomplete abortion, premature labour, intrauterine foetal death, and birth defects [3].

Therefore, the use of misoprostol for the prevention and treatment of gastric and duodenal ulcers is contraindicated in women who are or might be pregnant. Women of childbearing age must be recommended to use an adequate method of contraception (e.g. the contraceptive pill or an intrauterine device). Misoprostol is also contraindicated in breast-feeding mothers; it may cause adverse drug reactions (e.g. diarrhoea) in the child [3].

2.3 Off-label Use

Misoprostol is only licensed for oral administration for the prevention and treatment of peptic ulcers. For all indications in obstetrics and gynaecology, it is used as an off-label drug. What does "off-label" mean?

2.3.1 Off-label Use in General

Before a drug is licensed, its effectiveness and safety have to be proven and tested by the responsible legal authority, e.g. the Food and Drug Administration (FDA) in the United States or the Swiss Agency for Therapeutic Products in Switzerland, in preclinical and clinical studies [19].

With its license, each drug gets a so-called "label", which contains expert information about the approved indication(s), dose regimens (dosage, interval of application, etc.), patient population, as well as technical-pharmacological guidelines (e.g. duration of storability or the use of additional solvents). If a drug is used outside of one or more of the labelled prescriptions, it is said to be used "off-label". This means that the drug is administered without permission of the admission authority [20, 21].

In Switzerland, the use of off-label drugs is allowed. The legislation is contained in the *Schweizerisches Heilmittelgesetz (HMG Bundesgesetz vom 15. 12. 2000)*, which came into effect on 1st January, 2002 [20, 21].

When using an off-label drug, the physician and the pharmacist carry the responsibility for its prescription and application *(Art. 26 Abs. 1)*. They have to inform the patient at least orally about the use of off-label drugs and should be able to give a plausible explanation as to why they consider the use of the drug to be reasonable. They also have to inform the patient that health insurance is not obliged to pay for the off-label drug [20, 21].

The term "off-label use" has to be strictly separated from the term "unlicensed use", which means that the drug is not labelled by the responsible legal authority and its application is not allowed in the country. There are special cases, where the drug can be imported from other countries (where it is approved) [20, 21].

2.3.2 Off-label Use in Pregnancy

For different reasons, pharmaceutical companies are often not very ambitious about getting a license for the use of their drugs for obstetric indications. First, they would be obliged to conduct additional studies that prove the efficacy and safety of the drug in pregnant women, which is a time-consuming and also very expensive process. Secondly, they are afraid of possible legal and financial consequences, should any adverse drug reactions occur, which could be associated with their drug [21].

Therefore, the use of off-label drugs in obstetrics as well as in gynaecology, oncology, and paediatrics is a widespread phenomenon.

Some of the most frequently used off-label drugs in obstetrics are misoprostol (for the indications mentioned above), nifedipine for tocolysis, and betamethasone for the induction of foetal lung maturity in cases of imminent premature labour [21].

2.4 Aim of this Study

This work was carried out to pool and evaluate published data on the use of misoprostol in obstetrics since 1987, focussing the incidence of the most common ADR in mother and child, in order to evaluate the safety of misoprostol in the three main obstetrical indications (cervical ripening and labour induction, abortion induction, prevention and treatment of PPH). In addition, an attempt was made to describe the drug's efficacy within certain parameters of delivery (e.g. the caesarean-section rate).

Furthermore, this thesis aims to give an overview of the problems of off-label use in obstetrics, as well as general information about the characteristics of the drug misoprostol itself.

The implementation of our study was announced at the legal Swiss Agency for Therapeutic Products beforehand and submitted after conclusion for a closing statement and advice regarding a further approach.

3. Material and Methods

To pool and evaluate existing data on the efficacy and safety of misoprostol in its off-label use in obstetrics, the online database PubMed was searched for studies that had administered misoprostol to pregnant women for its three main obstetrical indications. Information on the included studies was summarised and further processed in an Excel database. In a second step, the observed adverse drug reactions in mothers and children and adverse events during birth were recorded and statistically evaluated.

3.1 Search Strategy in PubMed Database

First, the online database PubMed was searched for the following terms:

- misoprostol AND cervical ripening
- misoprostol AND induction AND labour
- misoprostol AND abortion AND induction
- misoprostol AND postpartum haemorrhage and hemorrhage

The primary search was started on 28.1.2011. The date of the latest search was 31.5.2011. In total, 2275 studies, conducted from 1987 to 2011, resulted.

The selection of the studies recorded in the analysis according to the following criteria left 647 includible studies.

3.2 Selection of Studies

3.2.1 Study Population

Cervical Ripening and Labour Induction

Women in the first or second trimester of pregnancy with an indication for cervical ripening prior to surgical evacuation of the uterus and women in the late second or third trimester of pregnancy with an indication for cervical ripening and/or labour induction at term.

Abortion Induction

Women in the first or second trimester of pregnancy with an indication for the induction of abortion after intrauterine foetal death, missed or incomplete abortion, or voluntary interruption of pregnancy (legally or illegally).

Prevention or Treatment of PPH

Women in the third trimester of pregnancy with an indication for the prevention of PPH or needing treatment of PPH.

The women included in the studies received treatment either by misoprostol alone, misoprostol in combination with oxytocin or other drugs (excluding mifepristone, trilostane, methotrexate, and nitric oxide), surgical termination, or mechanical methods (such as Foley catheter or Dilpan-S).

Misoprostol was administrated orally, vaginally, sublingually, buccally, rectally, or cervically.

Studies in women with prior caesarean section were also included in the analysis.

3.2.2 Study Designs

Randomised controlled trials (RCTs) were included as well as observational studies, controlled trials, retrospective analysis of RCTs, cohort studies (pro and retrospective), case-control studies, case series, and case reports.

Systematic reviews, meta-analyses, and Cochrane reviews found on PubMed were recorded in a separate chart, but were not included later in the analysis.

According to the guidelines of the Cochrane database, these types of studies are defined as follows:

Descriptive Studies
- **Case series**: "A study retrospectively reporting observations on a series of individuals, usually all receiving the same intervention, with no control group" [22].
- **Case report**: "A study reporting observations on a single individual" [22].
- **Observational studies:** "A study prospectively reporting observations on a series of individuals, usually all receiving the same intervention, with no control group" [22].
- **Case-control study**: "Compares people with a specific disease or outcome of interest (cases) to people from the same population without that disease or outcome (controls)" [22].
- **Cohort study**: "A defined group of people (cohort) is followed over time. The outcomes of people in subsets of this cohort are compared, to examine people who were exposed or not/different to a particular intervention" [22].

- Prospective: "Assembles participants and follows them into the future" [22].
- Retrospective ("historical"): "Identifies subjects from past records and follows them from the time of those records to the present" [22].

Experimental Studies
- **Controlled trial**: "Using quasi-randomisation or double-blinding, but randomisation was not mentioned" [22].
- **RCT:** "Randomisation by random numbers table or computer-generated random sequence" [22].

Secondary Studies
- **Cochrane database review**: "Systematic summaries of evidence of the effects of healthcare interventions" [22].
- **Systematic review**: "Uses systematic and explicit methods to identify, select, and critically appraise relevant research. A meta-analysis may or may not be used to analyse and summarise the results of the included studies" [22].
- **Meta-analysis:** "Use of statistical techniques in a systematic review to integrate the results of the included studies (sometimes misused as a synonym for systematic review, when the review includes a meta-analysis)" [22].

3.2.3 Language

Included were studies published in English, German, or French.

3.2.4 Excluded Studies

- Studies with other study designs than the ones mentioned above.
- Studies, where misoprostol was used in combination with other abortifacients, namely mifepristone, trilostane, methotrexate, or nitric oxide (NO).
- Studies in non-pregnant women (e.g. for softening of the cervix prior to hysteroscopy in post-menopausal women).
- Studies, where the full text was not available or was written in languages other than English, German, or French.
- Duplicates: Studies found on PubMed with two or more different search terms (e.g. with "misoprostol and cervical ripening" as well as with "misoprostol and labour induction").
- Studies listed under false indication (e.g. studies concerning cervical ripening prior to surgical abortion under "misoprostol and abortion induction" instead of "misoprostol and cervical ripening") were treated as duplicates and excluded.

3.3 Description and Analysis of the Included Studies

3.3.1 Database

The characteristics of the included studies were presented in three Excel charts, separated by the three main indications.

Each line in a chart represents a study. In the case of studies with more than one study group receiving medication with misoprostol, each group is depicted in a separate line. In the first step, only the data of women receiving misoprostol was included in the database. For the meta-analyses carried out later in the process, the necessary information about the other study groups was added, but only for the studies included in one or more of the meta-analyses.

The database was then divided into the following main sections, depicted in the columns of the chart:

Information about the selected Studies

This section contains information about the selected studies, including their PMID (as declared on PubMed), the original author, year of publication, study design, and whether the data was recorded pro or retrospectively. There is also a column containing information about the different regimens that were compared in the studies with more than one study group. Primary outcome is also recorded in a separate column.

Information about the Use of Misoprostol

This section concerns the use of misoprostol. The columns contain information about the detailed indication for which misoprostol was administered (e.g. cervical ripening prior to labour induction vs. cervical ripening prior to surgical termination), whether it was used alone or in combination with other methods (e.g. other drugs or surgical termination), whether it was combined with oxytocin or not, the mode of application of the drug, the maximum first single dose, the maximum number of dosages over 24 h, and the maximum dose administered in 24 h.

Additional Medication with Oxytocin or other Uterotonics

For the indication cervical ripening and labour induction the charts also list whether women were to receive additional oxytocin for the induction or augmentation of labour and the number of women that actually received this additional treatment; likewise for the indication prevention or treatment of PPH, where the charts show, whether the women received an additional uterotonic (e.g. oxytocin, ergometrine, or syntometrine).

Study Population

Two columns give information about the number of women in the study group and their trimesters of pregnancy.

An additional column in the chart for cervical ripening and/or labour induction contains the number of newborns included in the study group.

Maternal and neonatal Adverse Drug Reactions (ADR) and Delivery

Information about the observed ADR during study time was collected for all women included in the studies.

The first column shows whether ADR were measured or not. Further, the resulting groups of ADR were listed for each of the three indications, and the number of women suffering from these ADR was recorded in the column.

Incidences of serious maternal ADR, such as uterine rupture and maternal death, were evaluated separately.

Adverse events during childbirth were evaluated in the same manner for all three indications, and for indication cervical ripening and labour induction also the adverse reactions of the newborns.

Table 1: Evaluated parameters of maternal and neonatal adverse drug reactions and delivery

Group of ADR	Definition	Evaluated in indications		
		Cervical ripening and labour induction	Abortion induction	Prevention of PPH
Maternal ADR					
Gastrointestinal ADR	Nausea, vomiting and/or diarrhoea	Yes	Yes	Yes
Fever and/or shivering	Fever, hyperthermia, pyrexia, shivering, chills	Yes	Yes	Yes
Infection	Endometritis, chorioamnionitis, urinary-tract infection, PID, sepsis, puerperal sepsis, post-operative infection, infectious morbidity, wound infection	Yes	Yes	Yes
Maternal death		Yes	Yes	Yes
Other ADR	Abdominal discomfort, abruption of the placenta, acute anaemia, asthenia, blood-pressure alterations, breast tenderness, clot retention, confusion, cryptogenic stroke, disseminated intravascular coagulopathy (DIC), dizziness, eclamptic seizure, eclampsia, extremity cramping, fainting, fatigue, haematometra, (hot) flush, giddiness, glottal oedema, hypotension, hypertension, hypovolaemic shock, hypothermia, itching, malaise, misoprostol allergy, oliguria, palpitation, paraesthesia, postpartum uterine atony, preeclampsia, rapid pulse, rapid respiration, rash, redness, rigors, severe maternal morbidity,	Yes	Yes	Yes

	severe upper GI bleeding, severe postpartum anaemia, shortness of breath, systemic collapse, sweating, tachycardia, tetanic uterus, tiredness, unpleasant taste in the mouth, urinary frequency tenesmus, vaginal symptoms, vertigo, weakness, "other ADR", "ADR", "minor complications"			
Delivery				
Uterine contraction abnormalities without foetal heart-rate changes	Uterine tachysystolia (five or more contractions in 10 minutes for two consecutive 10-minute periods), hypersystolia (single contraction with a duration of more than 90 s), and hypertonus (single contraction with a duration of at least 2 minutes)	Yes	No	No
Hyperstimulation syndrome	Uterine contraction abnormalities with foetal heart-rate changes	Yes	No	No
Uterine dehiscence / rupture	Uterine rupture, dehiscence, perforation, utero-cervical laceration, intraoperative uterine damage	Yes	Yes	No
Genital or perineal trauma	Vagina or cervical laceration, perineal tear, intraoperative cervical damage	Yes	No	No
Mild or moderate bleeding	Vaginal bleeding, vaginal spotting; light, mild, scant, or moderate bleeding; metrorrhagie	Yes	Yes	No
Heavy bleeding, PPH	PPH (≥500 ml after vaginal birth, ≥1'000 after caesarean section, decrease in Hb of ≥10%), haemorrhage, heavy bleeding, severe bleeding, significant bleeding, blood loss requiring transfusion	Yes	Yes	Yes

Other intrapartum complications	Dystocia, placental abruption, precipitate labour/delivery	Yes	No	No
Caesarean section (CS)	Number of newborns delivered by CS, independent of exact cause	Yes	No	No

Neonatal ADR				
Apgar ≤6 at 5 min		Yes	No	No
Admission to NICU	Newborns admitted to neonatal intensive care unit (NICU), paediatrician, or nursery	Yes	No	No
Presence of signs of foetal distress	Meconium passage, nonreassuring FHR, abnormal FHR, nonreassuring foetal status, base excess >12, umbilical artery pH <7.16, cord pH <7.16, late decelerations, severe variable decelerations, foetal tachycardia, pathological CTG, "foetal distress"	Yes	No	No
Neonatal death		Yes	No	No
Other neonatal ADR	Asphyxia neonatorum, breathing difficulties, cord complications, hyperbilirubinaemia, hypoxia, hypoxic ischaemic encephalopathy, need for resuscitation, meconium aspiration, neonatal infection, neonatal sepsis, respiratory distress, respiratory difficulty, seizure, transient tachypnea, "other neonatal complications"	Yes	No	No

Serious adverse (drug) reactions (SAR), including uterine dehiscence or rupture and maternal death, were additionally depicted in a separate file for all three indications.

Meta-analyses

The last column shows the Cochrane reviews, other systematic reviews, and meta-analyses conducted by other authors, which included this study for a secondary analysis.

3.3.2 Analysed Aspects

In a first step, the focus of analysis was laid on the ADR observed in mothers and neonates and the outcome of birth after exposure to misoprostol. Data was analysed by different subgroups formed by focussing on different characteristics of the study conditions (e.g. indication, trimester of pregnancy, maximal dose of misoprostol, or mode of application). Serious adverse events, including uterine dehiscence or rupture and maternal death, were evaluated separately. Data from the included studies were coded and differentiated by several subgroups (Excel).

In this step of analysis, data from all types of studies was included.

In a second step, meta-analyses of RCT, comparing two different regimens of misoprostol or misoprostol vs. placebo or other drugs were used. If there were at least four studies that compared two different methods of using misoprostol or that compared the use of misoprostol to another treatment regimen, they were included in a meta-analysis. Because the different ADR were not registered in all studies, only the ones that were registered most frequently were analysed. If a study compared more than two groups (e.g. oral vs. vaginal vs. sublingual misoprostol), only the data from the groups compared in the other studies was taken for evaluation in the meta-analysis.

3.3.3 Statistical Methods

For discrete data (ADR), the relative frequencies were computed as well as the relative risk (RR random) with the corresponding 95% upper and lower confidence intervals (CI 95%). . The continuous parameters (such as max. dose) were described by mean and minimum/maximum. We conducted a meta-analysis of binary outcome data with the package "meta" in R (Guido Schwarzer (2010). meta: Meta-Analysis with R. R package version 1.6-1. http://CRAN.R-project.org/package=meta).

Data was tested for heterogeneity by the Mantel-Haenszel method and plotted in a forest plot and a funnel plot for the detection of publication bias.

A p-value < 0.05 was considered as statistically significant in all analyses.

4. Results

4.1 Overview

The primary search on PubMed resulted in 2275 studies. Of these studies, 647 fulfilled the inclusion criteria and were further analysed. Regarding the three main indications, there were 288 studies for cervical ripening and labour induction, 273 for abortion induction, and 86 for the prevention or treatment of PPH.

4.1.1 Studies

Table 2: References PubMed (1.1.80-31.5.2011)

	All results	Meta-analyses only	All, exclusively reviews	Used	RCT	Others
All						
Misoprostol (animal)	493	0	444			
Misoprostol (human)	3'090	59	2'275			
Pregnancy						
Misoprostol and pregnancy (animal)	38	0	32			
Misoprostol and pregnancy (human)	1'944	41	1'684			
Misoprostol and cervical ripening (human)	345	15	282			
Misoprostol and labour induction (human)	576	17	488			

Misoprostol and cervical ripening and labour induction (human)				288	218	70
Misoprostol and abortion (human)	1'121	18	974	273	116	157
Misoprostol and postpartum haemorrhage (human)	233	8	181	86	64	22
Pharmacokinetics						
Misoprostol and pharmacokinetics and human	91	0	60			

N = number of studies found on PubMed

Table 3: Selected studies and its main indications

	Cervical ripening and labour induction	Abortion induction	Prevention of PPH
Selected studies (n)	921	1'121	233
Included (n)	288	273	86
RCTs	218	116	64
Others	70	157	22
Excluded (n)	632	848	147
Other study design:			
- Guideline	19	25	39
- Review article	92	38	14
- Survey	9	27	7
- Monte Carlo	0	2	0
- Meta-analysis	32	18	8
- Pharmacokinetic	11	18	10
Nonpregnant women	37	9	0
Foreign language	48	59	12
Mifepristone	6	548	8
Trilostane	1	2	0
Methotrexate	0	69	0
Nitric oxide (NO)	3	0	0
Duplicates	291	0	0
Listed under false	78	26	48
Full text not available	5	7	1

N = number of studies

Table 4: Included studies: design and indications

	Cervical ripening and labour induction (N)	Abortion induction (N)	Prevention of PPH (N)
Included studies (n)	**288**	**273**	**86**
RCT (total)	218	116	64
Controlled trial	1	2	0
Retrospective analysis	3	0	2
Observational study	15	63	6
Prospective cohort	10	12	5
Pro and retrospective cohort study	3	2	0
Retrospective cohort	15	13	2
Case-control study	1	9	0
Case series	9	29	2
Case report	13	29	5

N = number of studies

For inclusion and exclusion criteria see chapter 3 "Material and Methods".

More detailed information about the characteristics of the included RCTs is shown in the appendix.

4.1.2 Women

Of all included studies, information about women receiving misoprostol was recorded and included in the Excel database. In this step of analysis, information about women receiving other treatment than misoprostol, e.g. the control group in an RCT, was not evaluated. The parameters listed in the following tables were analysed according to the three main obstetrical indications of misoprostol.

For all studies taken together, there were a total number of 52'379 women receiving misoprostol for the indication cervical ripening and/or labour induction, 42'056 for abortion induction, and 32'042 for the prevention or treatment of PPH.

Table 5: Included women

	Cervical ripening and labour induction		Abortion induction		Prevention of PPH	
Total women	n	%	N	%	n	%
Trimester of pregnancy						
Trimester 1 (week 0-12)	12'890	24.6	21'0	50.0	80	0.2
Trimester 2 (week 13-24)	9'226	17.6	14'6	34.7	821	2.6
Trimester 3 (week 25-40)	28'260	54.0	1	0.0	31'141	97.2
Detailed indication						
Only cervical ripening	23'197	(44.3)				
Only labour induction	7'166	(13.7)				
Cervical ripening and labour	20'984	(40.1)				
First-trimester abortion			20'3	(48.		
First and second-trimester abortion			4'91 1	(11. 7)		
Second-trimester abortion			14'6	(34.		
Second and third-trimester abortion			1'68 3	(4.0)		
Prevention of PPH					29'778	(92.9
Treatment of PPH					2'264	(7.1)

Misoprostol: Details on use						
Vaginal	25'356	(48.4)	24'228	(57.6)	45	(0.1)
Oral	10'744	(20.5)	4'400	(10.5)	23'314	(72.8)
Sublingual	3'030	(5.8)	5'386	(12.8)	4'667	(14.6)
Rectal	0	(0.0)	191	(0.0)	3'268	(10.2)
Misoprostol alone	29'066	(55.5)	37'405	(88.9)	27'421	(85.6)
Misoprostol in combination	23'313	(44.5)	4'651	(11.1)	4'621	(14.4)
With oxytocin	882	(1.7)	1'742	(4.1)		
Without oxytocin	51'497	(98.3)	40'314	(95.9)		
Additional oxytocin if necessary	21'818	(41.7)				
Additional oxytocin given	9'600	(18.3)				
With oxytocics*					4498	(14.0)
Without oxytocics					27'544	(86.0)
Additional oxytocics* if necessary					25'729	(80.3)
Additional oxytocics* given					3'266	(10.2)

* Oxytocin, syntometrine, ergometrine

Cervical ripening and labour induction includes all women treated with misoprostol at term for cervical ripening and induction of labour as well as women needing cervical preparation prior to surgical termination of pregnancy in the first or second trimester.

Abortion induction includes all women which terminated pregnancy medically in the first or second trimester. One single case report gave information about the termination of pregnancy in the 3rd trimester.

Prevention of PPH includes women who received misoprostol at term respectively after birth of the child for the prevention or treatment of PPH. The few cases of women in the first or second trimester were surgical terminations of pregnancy, where misoprostol was given with the intent to lower intraoperative blood loss.

4.2 Maternal Adverse Drug Reactions (ADR)

In a first process of analysis, data of all available studies was evaluated with the Excel database, separating the studies into three different groups according to the three main indications.

Data was processed by forming subgroups considering different aspects of the use of misoprostol and analysed by comparison of the different subgroups. Evaluated were the incidence of maternal ADR and the outcome of delivery for all indications, and additionally neonatal ADR for cervical ripening and labour induction.

4.2.1 Overview

A total of 47'274 women receiving misoprostol for the indication cervical ripening and/or labour induction, 40'741 for the induction of abortion and 32'012 for the prevention or treatment of PPH were observed for the ADR listed in table 6.

Table 6: Overview maternal ADR

	Cervical ripening and labour induction			Abortion induction			Prevention of PPH		
ADR	Total	With ADR	CI 95%	Total	With ADR	CI 95%	Total	With ADR	CI 95%
Gastrointestinal ADR	18'359	2'929 (16.0)	15.4 - 16.5	27'713	12'694 (45.8)	45.2 - 46.4	26'229	1'835 (7.0)	6.7 - 7.3
Fever and/or shivering	13'157	1'165 (8.9)	8.4 - 9.4	26'737	10'567 (39.5)	38.9 - 40.1	28'439	10'623 (37.4)	36.8 - 37.9
Infection*	11'768	561 (4.8)	4.4 - 5.2	7'128	285 (4.0)	3.6 - 4.5	1'041	19 (1.8)	1.2 - 2.8
Maternal death	52'379	4 (0.0)	0.0 - 0.0	42'056	3 (0.0)	0.0 - 0.0	32'042	21 (0.1)	0.0 - 0.1
Other maternal ADR	7'270	372 (5.1)	4.6 - 5.6	11'349	2'113 (18.6)	17.9 - 19.3	7'389	1'391 (18.8)	18.0 - 19.7

*(endometritis, chorioamnionitis, PID)

Data is n (%) of observed women.

4.2.2 Maternal ADR by Trimester of Pregnancy

More than half of the women requiring treatment with misoprostol for cervical ripening and labour induction (54.0%) were at term of pregnancy. Most of the women needing abortion induction were in the first or second trimester of pregnancy; only one case report documented a termination in the third trimester.

Most of the women receiving misoprostol for the prevention or treatment of PPH were at term (97.2%), the remaining few cases reported the attempt to lower intraoperative bleeding during the surgical termination of pregnancy.

To analyse whether the frequency of ADR after the intake of misoprostol had changed thorough pregnancy, the cases were separated according to trimester and indication.

A total of 12'890 women receiving misoprostol in the first trimester of pregnancy for the indication cervical ripening and/or labour induction and 21'020 for abortion induction were observed for the ADR listed in table 7. There were no women in the first trimester receiving misoprostol for the prevention or treatment of PPH.

Table 7: ADR first trimester of pregnancy

	Cervical ripening and labour induction			Abortion induction			All indications		
ADR	Total	With ADR	CI 95%	Total	With ADR	CI 95%	Total	With ADR	CI 95%
Gastrointestinal ADR	6'609	1'786 (27.0)	26.0 - 28.1	16'401	8'592 (52.4)	51.6 - 53.2	23'090	10'380 (45.0)	44.3 - 45.6
Fever and/or shivering	4'828	680 (14.1)	13.1 - 15.1	15'289	5'801 (37.9)	37.2 - 38.7	20'197	6'484 (32.1)	31.5 - 32.8
Infection *	3'711	9 (0.2)	0.1 - 0.5	4'684	197 (4.2)	3.7 - 4.8	8'395	206 (2.5)	2.1 - 2.8
Maternal death	12'890	0 (0.0)	0.0 - 0.0	21'020	1 (0.0)	0.0 - 0.0	33'990	1 (0.0)	0.0 - 0.0
Other ADR	2'179	210 (9.6)	8.5 - 10.9	6'750	1'264 (18.7)	17.8 - 19.7	8'929	1'474 (16.5)	15.8 - 17.3

*(endometritis, chorioamnionitis, PID...)

Data is n (%) of observed women.

A total of 9'226 women receiving misoprostol in the second trimester of pregnancy for the indication cervical ripening and/or labour induction and 14'613 for abortion induction were observed for the ADR listed in table 8. There were no women in the second trimester receiving misoprostol for the prevention or treatment of PPH.

Table 8: ADR second trimester of pregnancy

ADR	Cervical ripening and labour induction Total	With ADR	CI 95%	Abortion induction Total	With ADR	CI 95%	All indications Total	With ADR	CI 95%
Gastrointestinal ADR	2'237	4 (0.2)	0.1 - 0.5	8'876	3'073 (34.6)	33.6 - 35.6	11'113	3'077 (27.7)	26.9 - 28.5
Fever and/or	2'218	3 (0.1)	0.0 - 0.4	9'772	4'186 (42.8)	41.9 - 43.8	11'990	4'189 (34.9)	34.1 - 35.8
Infection *	2'450	12 (0.5)	0.3 - 0.9	1'897	71 (3.7)	3.0 - 4.7	4'347	83 (1.9)	1.5 - 2.4
Maternal death	9'226	0 (0.0)	0.0 - 0.0	14'613	1 (0.0)	0.0 - 0.0	23'839	1 (0.0)	0.0 - 0.0
Other ADR	2'218	1 (0.0)	0.0 - 0.3	3'228	641 (19.9)	18.5 - 21.3	5'446	642 (11.8)	11.0 - 12.7

* (endometritis, chorioamnionitis, PID)

Data is n (%) of observed women.

A total of 28'260 women receiving misoprostol in the third trimester of pregnancy for the indication cervical ripening and/or labour induction and 31'141 for the prevention or treatment of PPH were observed for the ADR listed in table 9. There were no women in the third trimester receiving misoprostol for abortion induction.

Table 9: ADR third trimester of pregnancy

	Cervical ripening and labour induction			Prevention of PPH			All indications		
ADR	Total	With ADR	CI 95%	Total	With ADR	CI 95%	Total	With ADR	CI 95%
Gastrointestinal ADR	8'807	1'060 (12.0)	11.4 - 12.7	25'328	1'804 (7.1)	6.8 - 7.4	34'135	2864 (8.4)	8.1 - 8.7
Fever and/or	6'058	445 (7.3)	6.7 - 8.0	27'538	10'496 (38.1)	37.5 - 38.7	33'596	10941 (32.6)	32.1 - 33.1
Infection *	4'820	521 (10.8)	10.0 - 11.7	664	12 (1.8)	1.0 - 3.1	5'484	533 (9.7)	9.0 - 10.5
Maternal death	28'260	4 (0.0)	0.0 - 0.0	31'141	11 (0.0)	0.0 - 0.1	59'401	15 (0.0)	0.0 - 0.0
Other ADR	2'873	161 (5.6)	4.8 - 6.5	6'945	1'277 (18.4)	17.5 - 19.3	9'818	1438 (14.6)	14.0 - 15.4

*(endometritis, chorioamnionitis, PID)

Data is n (%) of observed women.

The most frequently observed ADR in all trimesters and for all indications were gastrointestinal ADR (including nausea, vomiting, and diarrhoea) and fever and/or shivering. Fever and shivering occurred in about one third of the women in all trimesters, whereas gastrointestinal ADR were much more frequent in women in the second trimester of pregnancy (up to 45% of the women suffered them) but less common in the third trimester, where they occurred in only 8.4% of the patients.

4.2.3 Maternal ADR by Indication

Most of the women summarised under the indication cervical ripening and/or labour induction received misoprostol for cervical ripening with or without labour induction (44.3% and 40.1 % respectively). Women needing only cervical ripening include cases of cervical ripening prior to surgical termination as well as women at term receiving another drug for the induction of labour after ripening of the cervix with misoprostol or without any medication for induction after cervical ripening. Therefore, this group is quite heterogeneous compared to the two others that include also labour induction, which is usually conducted at term regarding characteristics such as trimester of pregnancy or the given dose of misoprostol.

For the indication abortion induction, the most frequent reason for the administration of misoprostol was induction of abortion in the first trimester of pregnancy (48.4 %). 34.8% of the women needed the induction of abortion in the second trimester. There was one single case of abortion induction in the third trimester. The remaining 11.7% aborted either in the first or second trimester, which means that it was not clear from the study report, in which trimester the women were.

Most of the women (92.9%) received misoprostol for the prevention of PPH; the remaining 7.1% needed treatment of PPH.

To assess whether the frequency of occurring ADR varies between the different indications, they were evaluated separately for each of the three main indications.

23'197 women receiving misoprostol only for cervical ripening, 7'166 only for labour induction, and 20'984 for both indications were observed for the ADR listed in table 10.

Table 10: ADR in women with indication cervical ripening and/or labour induction

	Only cervical ripening			Only labour induction			Cervical ripening and labour induction		
ADR	Total	With ADR	CI 95%	Total	With ADR	CI 95%	Total	With ADR	CI 95%
Gastrointestinal ADR	9'680	1'882 (19.4)	18.7 - 20.2	1'413	288 (20.4)	18.4 -	7'266	759 (10.4)	9.8 - 11.2
Fever and/or shivering	7'099	720 (10.1)	9.5 - 10.9	1'408	271 (19.2)	17.3 -	4'650	174 (3.7)	3.2 - 4.3
Infection*	6'717	37 (0.6)	0.4 - 0.8	299	37 (12.4)	9.1 - 16.6	4'752	487 (10.2)	9.4 - 11.1
Maternal death	23'197	0 (0.0)	0.0 - 0.0	7'166	2 (0.0)	0.0 - 0.1	20'984	2 (0.0)	0.0 - 0.0
Other ADR	4'543	211 (4.6)	4.1 - 5.3	694	28 (4.0)	2.8 - 5.8	2'033	133 (6.5)	5.5 - 7.7

*(endometritis, chorioamnionitis, PID)

Data is n (%) of observed women.

20'365 women receiving misoprostol for first and 14'643 for second-trimester abortions were observed for the ADR listed in table 11.

Table 11: ADR in women with indication abortion induction

	First trimester abortion			Second trimester abortion		
ADR	Total	With ADR	CI 95%	Total	With ADR	CI 95%
Gastrointestinal ADR	16'155	8'624 (53.4)	52.6 - 54.2	8'876	3'073 (34.6)	33.6 - 35.6
Fever and/or shivering	15'142	5'768 (38.1)	37.3 - 38.9	9'802	4'190 (42.7)	41.8 - 43.7
Infection	4'188	51 (1.2)	0.9 - 1.6	1'897	71 (3.7)	3.0 - 4.7
Maternal death	20'365	1 (0.0)	0.0 - 0.0	14'643	1 (0.0)	0.0 - 0.0
Other ADR	6'486	1'285 (19.8)	18.9 - 20.8	3'228	641 (19.9)	18.5 - 21.3

*(endometritis, chorioamnionitis, PID)

Data is n (%) of observed women.

29'778 women receiving misoprostol for the prevention of PPH were observed for the ADR listed in table 12.

Table 12: Maternal ADR in women with indication prevention of PPH

	Prevention of PPH		
ADR	Total	With ADR	CI 95%
Gastrointestinal ADR	24'291	1'427 (5.9)	5.6 - 6.2
Fever and/or shivering	26'386	8'344 (31.6)	31.1 - 32.2
Infection (endometritis, chorioamnionitis, PID)	1'037	19 (1.8)	1.2 - 2.8
Maternal death	29'778	15 (0.1)	0.0 - 0.1
Other ADR	n. e.		

Data is n (%) of observed women.

4.2.4 Maternal ADR by different Modes of Application of Misoprostol

The frequency of the different modes of application varies in the three main indications. For the indications cervical ripening and labour induction as well as for abortion induction, vaginal application was most frequently used (48 and 58% respectively) in contrast to the prevention and treatment of PPH, where misoprostol was administered orally in the majority of cases (73%). To analyse whether the mode of application influences the frequency of ADR, data was compared according to oral, vaginal, sublingual, rectal, or other modes of application.

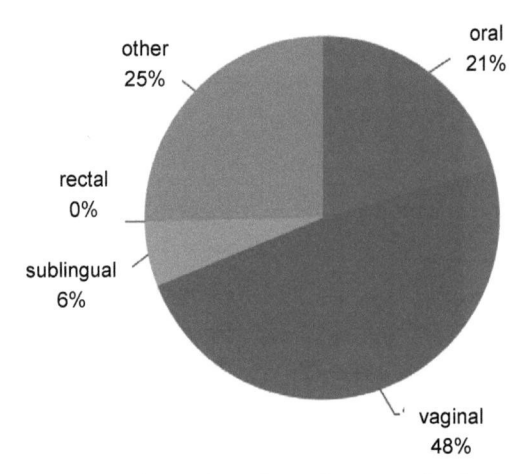

other 25%
oral 21%
rectal 0%
sublingual 6%
vaginal 48%

Figure 1: Mode of application for cervical ripening and labour induction

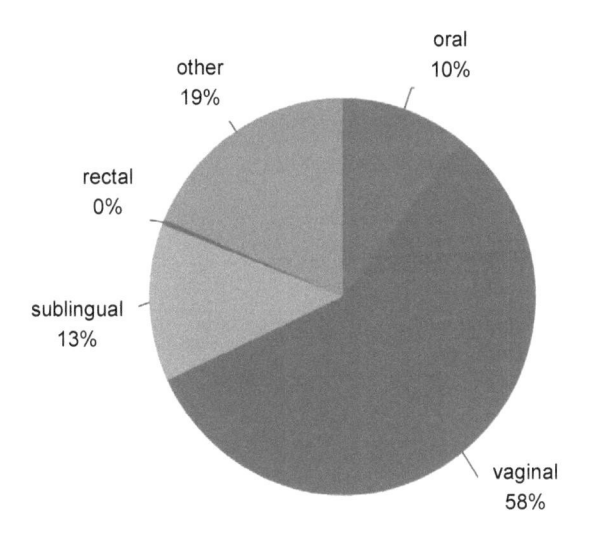

Figure 2: Mode of application for indication abortion induction

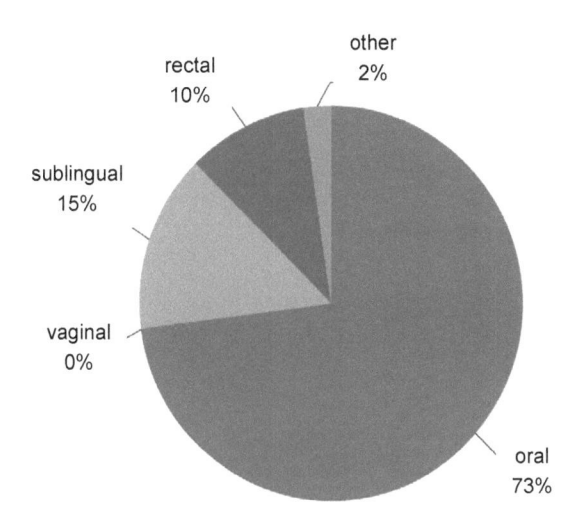

Figure 3: Mode of application for indication prevention or treatment of PPH

After oral application of misoprostol, 10'744 women with the indication cervical ripening and/or labour induction, 4'400 with abortion induction, and 23'314 with the prevention or treatment of PPH were observed for the ADR listed in table 13.

Table 13: Maternal ADR: oral application

	Cervical ripening and labour induction			Abortion induction			Prevention of PPH		
ADR	Total	With ADR	CI 95%	Total	With	CI 95%	Total	With ADR	CI 95%
Gastrointestinal ADR	6'665	1'396 (20.9)	20.0 - 21.9	2'706	878 (32.4)	30.7 - 34.2	20'766	1'193 (5.7)	5.4 - 6.1
Fever and/or shivering	3'208	507 (15.8)	14.6 - 17.1	2'560	440 (17.2)	15.8 - 18.7	21'471	6'736 (31.4)	30.8 - 32.0
Infection*	2'738	122 (4.5)	3.7 - 5.3	732	15 (2.0)	1.2 - 3.4	489	2 (0.4)	0.1 - 1.5
Maternal death	10'744	0 (0.0)	0.0 - 0.0	4'400	2 (0.0)	0.0 - 0.2	23'314	14 (0.1)	0.0 - 0.1
Other ADR	2'631	148 (5.6)	4.8 - 6.6	622	41 (6.6)	4.9 - 8.8	4'754	1'076 (22.6)	21.5 - 23.8

* (endometritis, chorioamnionitis, PID)

Data is n (%) of observed women.

After vaginal application of misoprostol, 25'356 women with the indication cervical ripening and/or labour induction and 24'228 with abortion induction were observed for the ADR listed in table 14.

Table 14: Maternal ADR: vaginal application

	Cervical ripening and labour induction			Abortion induction		
ADR	Total	With ADR	CI 95%	Total	With ADR	CI 95%
Gastrointestinal ADR	7'329	887 (12.1)	11.4 - 12.9	15'684	7'820 (49.9)	49.1 - 50.6
Fever and/or shivering	5'473	403 (7.4)	6.7 - 8.1	14'901	7'004 (47.0)	46.2 - 47.8
Infection*	4'342	366 (8.4)	7.6 - 9.3	5'202	94 (1.8)	1.5 - 2.2
Maternal death	25'356	4	0.0 - 0.0	24'228	1	0.0 - 0.0
Other ADR	2'631	142 (5.4)	4.6 - 6.3	7'389	1'529 (20.7)	19.8 - 21.6

*(endometritis, chorioamnionitis, PID)

Data is n (%) of observed women.

The evaluation of maternal ADR after sublingual and rectal administration of misoprostol is shown in the appendix.

When ADR in all indications were compared by mode of application, gastrointestinal ADR were more frequently observed after sublingual and vaginal application (41.4% CI 95%: 40.5-42.4 and 37.8% CI 95%: 37.1-38.4 respectively) than after oral or rectal application (11.5% CI 95%: 11.1-11.9 and 10.1% CI 95%: 8.8-11.6 respectively). Fever and shivering were more common after sublingual application (50.5% CI 95%: 49.6-51.5) than after vaginal (36.3% CI 95%: 35.6-36.9), oral (28.2% CI 95%: 27.7-28.7) and rectal (39.6% CI 95%: 37.4-41.8) application.

4.2.5 Maternal ADR by different Doses

There was a great variation of applied doses also within the same application mode which made the evaluation of the influence of the administered dose on the ADR in mother and child and the outcome of pregnancy extremely difficult. The first single dose ranged from 10 to 6'600 µg (both of the cases concerned cervical ripening and labour induction); the maximal dose administered in 24 h ranged from 25 to 6'600 µg (also both for cervical ripening and labour induction).

To evaluate whether the frequency of ADR depends on the dose applied in 24 hours, the data was divided into a low and a high-dose group. The division was made according to the frequency of women used a specific dose For this evaluation only the oral and the vaginal application modes were considered.

4'608 women observed for the ADR listed in table 15 received ≤ 300 µg oral misoprostol for cervical ripening and/or labour induction, 6'136 received > 300 µg per day.

Table 15: Maternal ADR: ≤ 300 µg vs. > 300 µg misoprostol

	≤ 300 µg/24 h			> 300 µg/24 h		
ADR	Total	With ADR	CI 95%	Total	With ADR	CI 95%
Gastrointestinal ADR	2'620	609 (23.3)	21.7-24.9	4'045	787 (19.5)	18.3-20.7
Fever and/or shivering	689	55 (8.0)	6.2-10.2	2'519	452 (17.9)	16.5-19.5
Infection*	1'489	74 (5.0)	4.0-6.2	1'249	48 (3.8)	2.9-5.1
Maternal death	4'608	0 (0.0)	0.0-0.1	6'136	0 (0.0)	0.0-0.1
Other ADR	518	98 (18.9)	15.8-22.5	999	50 (5.0)	3.8-6.5

*(endometritis, chorioamnionitis, PID)

Data is n (%) of observed women.

16'877 women observed for the ADR listed in table 16 received ≤ 200 µg vaginal misoprostol for cervical ripening and/or labour induction, 28'784 received > 200 µg per day.

Table 16: Maternal ADR: ≤ 200 µg vs. > 200 µg misoprostol

	≤ 200 µg/24 h			> 200 µg/24 h		
ADR	Total	With ADR	CI 95%	Total	With ADR	CI 95%
Gastrointestinal ADR	4'290	450 (10.5)	9.6-11.4	3'039	437 (14.4)	13.2-15.7
Fever and/or shivering	3'408	121 (3.6)	3.0-4.2	2'065	282 (13.7)	12.2-15.2
Infection*	3'359	331 (9.9)	8.9-10.9	983	35 (3.6)	2.6-4.9
Maternal death	16'877	4 (0.0)		28'784	0 (0.0)	0.0-0.0
Other ADR	1'334	42 (3.1)	2.3-4.2	1'297	100 (7.7)	6.4-9.3

*(endometritis, chorioamnionitis, PID)

Data is n (%) of observed women.

4.2.6 Maternal ADR with Misoprostol alone vs. in Combination with Oxytocin

Most of the studies in all three indications used misoprostol alone (55.5% for cervical ripening and labour induction, 88.9% for abortion induction, and 85.6% for the prevention or treatment of PPH). The reason for the lower percentage of misoprostol alone for the indication cervical ripening was the combination with surgery for first and second-trimester abortions. Oxytocin in combination with misoprostol was routinely given only in few cases, but administered in addition to misoprostol when necessary in about 10% of the cases for the indications cervical ripening and labour induction and the prevention or treatment of PPH, but not for abortion induction.

To assess whether the additional administration of oxytocin with misoprostol influences the frequency of ADR in the mother, the data of women receiving misoprostol alone was compared with the data of women receiving both drugs in combination.

After medication with misoprostol alone for cervical ripening and labour induction, 29'066 women were observed, 37'497 were observed for abortion induction, and 27'014 for the prevention or treatment of PPH for the ADR listed in table 17.

Table 17: Maternal ADR with misoprostol alone

	Cervical ripening and labour induction			Abortion induction			Prevention of PPH		
ADR	Total	With ADR	CI 95%	Total	With ADR	CI 95%	Total	With ADR	CI 95%
Gastrointestinal ADR	8'207	978 (11.9)	11.2 - 12.6	25'862	12'220	46.6 - 47.9	23'661	1'518 (6.4)	6.1 - 6.7
Fever and/or shivering	5'541	374 (6.7)	6.1 - 7.4	25'266	9'911 (39.2)	38.6 - 39.8	24'510	8'518 (34.8)	34.2 - 35.4
Infection*	4'995	506 (10.1)	9.3 - 11.0	6'999	271 (3.9)	3.4 - 4.3	487	2 (0.4)	0.1 - 1.5
Maternal death	29'066	4 (0.0)	0.0 - 0.0	37'497	3 (0.0)	0.0 - 0.0	27'014	15 (0.1)	0.0 - 0.1
Other ADR	2'401	63 (2.6)	2.1 - 3.3	10'658	2'037 (19.1)	18.4 - 19.9	5'556	1'293 (23.3)	22.2 - 24.4

*(endometritis, chorioamnionitis, PID)

Data is n (%) of observed women.

882 women were observed for the ADR listed in table 18 after medication with misoprostol in combination with oxytocin for cervical ripening and labour induction, 1'742 for abortion induction, and 4'498 for the prevention or treatment of PPH.

Table 18: Maternal ADR with misoprostol in combination with oxytocin

	Cervical ripening and labour induction			Abortion induction			Prevention of PPH		
ADR	Total	With ADR	CI 95%	Total	With ADR	CI 95%	Total	With ADR	CI 95%
Gastrointestinal ADR	278	21 (7.6)	5.0 - 11.3	1'217	336 (27.6)	25.2 - 30.2	2'157	234 (10.8)	9.6 - 12.2
Fever and/or shivering	200	4 (2.0)	0.8 - 5.0	1'251	538 (43.0)	40.3 - 45.8	3'518	1'865 (53.0)	51.4 - 54.7
Infection*	100	17 (17.0)	10.9 - 25.5	105	9 (8.6)	4.6 - 15.5	550	17 (3.1)	1.9 - 4.9
Maternal death	882	0 (0.0)	0.0 - 0.4	1'742	0 (0.0)	0.0 - 0.2	4'498	5 (0.1)	0.0 - 0.3
Other ADR	223	40 (17.9)	13.5 - 23.5	79	18 (22.8)	14.9 - 33.2	1'375	19 (1.4)	0.9 - 2.1

*(endometritis, chorioamnionitis, PID)

Data is n (%) of observed women.

93'577 women receiving medication with misoprostol alone were compared to 7'122 women receiving misoprostol in combination with oxytocin for the ADR listed in table 19. Medication with misoprostol was given for all three main indications.

Table 19: Comparison of misoprostol alone vs. misoprostol in combination with oxytocin in all indications

	Misoprostol alone			Misoprostol with oxytocin		
ADR	Total	With ADR	CI 95%	Total	With ADR	CI 95%
Gastrointestinal ADR	57'730	14'716 (25.5)	25.1 - 25.8	3'652	591 (16.2)	15.0 - 17.4
Fever and/or shivering	55'317	18'803 (34.0)	33.6 - 34.4	4'969	2'407 (48.4)	47.1 - 49.8
Infection*	12'481	779 (6.2)	5.8 - 6.7	755	43 (5.7)	4.3 - 7.6
Maternal death	93'577	22 (0.0)	0.0 - 0.0	7'122	5 (0.1)	0.0 - 0.2
Other ADR	18'615	3'393 (18.2)	17.7 - 18.8	1'677	77 (4.6)	3.7 - 5.7

*(endometritis, chorioamnionitis, PID)

Data is n (%) of observed women.

4.2.7 Maternal ADR by Evaluation of RCTs only

Regarding data taken only from RCTs, 27'223 women with the indication cervical ripening and/or labour induction, 19'843 for abortion induction and 29'117 for the prevention or treatment of PPH were observed for the ADR listed in table 20.

Table 20: Maternal ADR only in RCTs

ADR	Cervical ripening and labour induction			Abortion induction			Prevention of PPH		
	Total	With ADR	CI 95%	Total	With ADR	CI 95%	Total	With ADR	CI 95%
Gastrointestinal ADR	12'441	2'273 (18.3)	17.6 - 19.0	16'623	7'564 (45.5)	44.7 - 46.3	23'567	1'491 (6.3)	6.0 - 6.6
Fever and/or shivering	8'921	1'016 (11.4)	10.7 - 12.1	15'603	5'789 (37.1)	36.3 - 37.9	25'715	9'482 (36.9)	16.3 - 37.5
Infection*	5'426	504 (9.3)	8.5 - 10.1	2'469	42 (1.7)	1.3 - 2.3	1'037	19 (1.8)	1.2 - 2.8
Maternal death	27'223	2 (0.0)	0.0 - 0.0	19'843	1 (0.0)	0.0 - 0.0	29'117	11 (0.0)	0.0 - 0.1
Other ADR	3'832	344 (9.0)	8.1 - 9.9	3'563	772 (21.7)	20.3 - 23.1	6'298	984 (15.6)	14.7 - 16.5

*(endometritis, chorioamnionitis, PID)

Data is n (%) of observed women.

4.3 Maternal Serious Adverse (Drug) Reactions (SAR)

Serious adverse (drug) reactions namely dehiscence, perforation or rupture of the uterus, and maternal death that occurred during the studies or have been described in case reports were separately evaluated. They are listed in tables 21 - 25.

Table 21: Uterine rupture in women treated with misoprostol for cervical ripening and labour induction

Author, Year	Study design	Indication	Additional oxytocin	Mode of application	Max. dose /24 h (µg)	Type of maternal serious adverse reaction (SAR)	Total / with SAR
Abdul, M. A. 2007	RCT	Cervical ripening and labour induction	No	Vaginal	200	Uterine rupture	34 / 1
Afolabi, B. B. 2005	RCT	Cervical ripening and labour induction	i.n.	Vaginal	100	Uterine rupture	50 / 2
Berghahn, L. 2001	Case report	Cervical ripening prior to second-trimester abortion	No	Vaginal and buccal	400	Uterine rupture	1 / 1
Blanchette, H. A. 1999	Cohort study	Cervical ripening and labour induction	i.n.	Vaginal	275	Uterine rupture	145 / 4

Edwards, D. 1994	Observational study	Cervical ripening prior to first and second-trimester abortion	No	Oral	600	Uterine perforation	595 / 1
Goldberg, A. B. 2005	RCT	Cervical ripening prior to first-trimester abortion	No	Vaginal	400	Uterine perforation	41 / 1
Has, R. 2002	RCT	Cervical ripening and labour induction	i.n.	Vaginal	75	Uterine rupture	58 / 1
Hill, D. A. 2000	Cohort study	Cervical ripening and labour induction	No	Vaginal	300	Uterine dehiscence (1), uterine rupture (3)	48 / 4
Majoko, F. 2002	RCT	Labour induction	i.n.	Vaginal	200	Uterine rupture	63 / 2
Majoko, F. 2002	Case report	Labour induction	No	Vaginal	100	Uterine rupture	1 / 1
Majoko, F. 2002	Case report	Labour induction	Yes	Vaginal	100	Uterine rupture	1 / 1
Mazzone, M. E. 2006	Case report	Labour induction	Yes	Vaginal	25	Uterine rupture	1 / 1

Mittal, S. 2011	RCT	Cervical ripening prior to first-trimester abortion	No	Vaginal	400	Uterine perforation	295 / 2
Nucatola, D. 2008	Case series	Cervical ripening prior to second-trimester abortion	No	Vaginal or buccal	400	Uterine perforation	6'620 / 3
Oppe-gaard, K. S. 2004	RCT	Cervical ripening prior to first-trimester abortion	No	Oral	200	Uterine perforation	275 / 1
Poon, L. C. 2007	Cohort study	Cervical ripening prior to second-trimester abortion	No	Vaginal	600	Intraoperative uterine damage	9 / 1
Roberts, L. M. 2007	Case series	Labour induction	i.n.	Vaginal	100	Uterine rupture	1'998 / 2
Sciscione, A. C. 2001	RCT	Cervical ripening	i.n.	Vaginal	300	Uterine rupture	53 / 1
Sciscione, A. C. 1998	Case report	Cervical ripening	No	Vaginal	100	Uterine perforation after previous CS	1 / 1
Singh, B. M. 2005	Case report	Labour induction	No	Vaginal	50	Uterocervical laceration	1 / 1

| Szczesny, W. 2006 | Case series | Cervical ripening and labour induction | i.n. | Vaginal | 100 | Uterine rupture after previous CS | 136 / 1 |
| Wing, D. A. 2004 | RCT | Cervical ripening and labour induction | i.n. | Oral | 600 | Uterine rupture | 110 / 1 |

i.n.: if necessary

Data is n of observed women.

Table 22: Uterine rupture in women treated with misoprostol for abortion induction

Author, Year	Study design	Indication	Additional oxytocin	Mode of application	Max. dose /24 h (µg)	Type of maternal serious adverse reaction (SAR)	Total / with SAR
Al-Hussaini, T. K. 2001	Case report	Second-trimester abortion	Yes	Vaginal	200	Uterine rupture	1 / 1
Autry, A. M. 2002	Cohort study	Second-trimester abortion	No	?[1]	?[1]	Uterine rupture	125 / 1
Blohm, F. 2005	RCT	First-trimester abortion	No	Vaginal	400	Uterine perforation after following D&C	64 / 1
Chen, M. 1999	Case report	Second-trimester abortion after previous CS	No	Vaginal	200	Uterine dehiscence of scarred uterus	1 / 1
Coelho, H. L. 1993	Case series	First and second-trimester abortion	No	?[1]	?[1]	Uterine perforation	444 / 1
Coelho, H. L. 1994	Case series	First and second trimester abortion	No	Oral, vaginal	?[1]	Uterine perforation	3 / 3
Costa, S. H. 1993	Case series	First and second-trimester abortion	No	Oral, vaginal	?[1]	Uterine perforation after surgical curettage	458 / 6

Daskalakis, G. 2005	Case report	Second-trimester abortion after previous CS	No	Oral, vaginal	800	Uterine rupture of the scarred uterus	1 / 1
Daskalakis, G. J. 2005	Case-control study	Second-trimester abortion after previous CS	No	Oral, vaginal	2'400	Uterine rupture	216 / 1
Dickinson, J. E. 2009	Case series	Second-trimester abortion	No	Vaginal	1'600	Uterine rupture	1'066 / 1
Edwards, R. K. 2005	Cohort study	Second-trimester abortion	No	Vaginal	1'600	Uterine rupture	47 / 1
Fawzy, M. 2010	Case-control study	Second-trimester abortion	No	Vaginal	800	Silent uterine rupture	31 / 1
Lialios, G. 2006	Case report	First-trimester abortion	No	Vaginal	800	Uterine rupture of the scarred uterus	1 / 1
Low, Y. S. 2009	Case report	Second-trimester abortion	No	Oral	1'200	Uterine rupture	1 / 1
Nayki, U. 2005	Case report	Second-trimester abortion after previous CS	No	Vaginal	800	Uterine rupture of the scarred uterus	1 / 1
Naz, S. 2007	Observational study	First and second-trimester abortion	i.n.	Vaginal	1'200	Uterine rupture	200 / 1

[1] not mentioned in study report
[2] i.n.: if necessary

Table 23: Maternal death in women treated with misoprostol for cervical ripening and labour induction

Author, Year	Study design	Indication	Additional oxytocin	Mode of application	Max. dose /24 h (µg)	Type of maternal serious adverse reaction (SAR)	Total / with SAR
Daisley, H., Jr. 2000	case report	Labour induction	No	Vaginal	50	Maternal death after uterine rupture with hypovolaemic shock	1 / 1
Ezechi, O. C. 2004	case series	Cervical ripening and labour induction	i.n.[1]	Vaginal	200	Maternal death after uterine rupture	339 / 1
Tukur, J. 2007	RCT	Labour induction after eclampsia	No	Vaginal	100	Maternal death	25 / 1
Wing, D. A. 1996	RCT	Cervical ripening and labour induction	i.n.[1]	Vaginal	100 or 200[2]	Maternal death after amniotic fluid embolism	520 / 1

[1] if necessary
[2] not mentioned in study report, in which dose group the case of maternal death occurred

Data is n of observed women.

Table 24: Maternal death in women treated with misoprostol for abortion induction

Author, Year	Study design	Indication	Mode of application	Max. dose /24 h (µg)	Type of maternal serious adverse reaction (SAR)	Total / with SAR
Carbonell, J. L. 2008	RCT	Second-trimester abortion	Vaginal	2'000	Maternal death due to septic shock after surgical abortion	105 / 1
Daisley, H., Jr. 2000	Case report	First-trimester abortion	Oral	?[1]	Maternal death after septic and hypovolaemic shock	1 / 1
Henriques, A. 2007	Case report	Abortion induction	Oral	1'200	Multiorgan failure and death	1 / 1

[1] not mentioned in study report

Data is n of observed women.

Table 25: Maternal death in women treated with misoprostol for prevention of PPH

Author, Year	Study design	Indication	Misoprostol combined with…	Mode of application	Max. dose /24 h (µg)	Type of maternal serious adverse reaction (SAR)	Total / with SAR
Blum, J. 2010	RCT	Treatment of PPH	After failed oxytocin prophylaxis	Sublingual	800	Maternal death after DIC	407 / 1
Gulmezoglu, A. M. 2001	RCT	Prevention of PPH	Additional oxytocics if necessary	Oral	600	Maternal death	9'225 / 2
Hofmeyr, G. J. 2004	RCT	Treatment of PPH	Standard oxytocics (oxytocin and/or syntometrine)	Oral, sublingual and rectal	1'000	Maternal death	117 / 3
Hoj, L. 2005	RCT	Prevention of PPH	Additional oxytocics if necessary	Sublingual	600	Maternal death	330 / 1
Rajbhandari, S. 2010	Case series	Prevention of PPH		Oral	600	Maternal death	13'969 / 10
Walraven G. 2005	RCT	Prevention of PPH	Additional oxytocics if necessary	Oral	600	Maternal death	630 / 2
Widmer, M. 2010	RCT	Treatment of PPH	Standard uterotonic (mostly oxytocin)	Sublingual	600	Maternal death	704 / 2

Data is n of observed women.

4.4 Delivery

4.4.1 Overview

A total of 47'274 women with the indication cervical ripening and/or labour induction were observed for the events during delivery listed in table 26. For abortion induction, a total of 40'741 women was observed, and for prevention or treatment of PPH a total of 32'012.

Table 26: Maternal events during delivery

Event	Cervical ripening and labour induction Total	With event	CI 95%	Abortion induction Total	With event	CI 95%	Prevention of PPH Total	With event	CI 95%
Uterine contraction abnormalities without FHRch*	20'283	3'214 (15.8)	15.3 - 16.4	n. e.			n. e.		
Hyperstimulation syndrome	18'892	1'342 (7.1)	6.7 - 7.5	n. e.			n. e.		
Other intrapartum complications	4'029	65 (1.6)	1.3 - 2.1	n. e.			n. e.		
Uterine dehiscence or	11'303	36 (0.3)	0.2 - 0.4	2'514	14 (0.6)	0.3 - 0.9	n. e.		
Genital trauma	5'708	372 (6.5)	5.9 - 7.2	n. e.			n. e.		
Mild or moderate bleeding	8'216	1'898 (23.1)	22.2 - 24.0	4'672	3'701 (79.2)	78.0 - 80.4	n. e.		
Heavy bleeding or PPH	23'601	848 (3.6)	3.4 - 3.8	17'272	1'576 (9.1)	8.7 - 9.6	27'249	4'323 (15.9)	15.4 - 16.3
Caesarean section	27'537	5'967 (21.7)	21.2 - 22.2	n. e.			n. e.		

*Foetal heart-rate changes
n.e.: not evaluated
Data is n (%) of observed women.

4.4.2 Delivery Outcome by Trimester of Pregnancy

To analyse whether the outcome of pregnancy changes depending on the trimester of pregnancy, data was regarded by separating the cases according to trimester and indication.

Of the women in the first trimester of pregnancy, 12'890 with the indication cervical ripening and/or labour induction and 21'020 with the indication abortion induction were observed for the events during delivery listed in table 27.

Table 27: Delivery outcome in the first trimester of pregnancy

	Cervical ripening and labour induction			Abortion induction		
Event	Total	With event	CI 95%	Total	With event	CI 95%
Hyperstimulation syndrome	n. e.			n. e.		
Uterine dehiscence or rupture	n. e.			n. e.		
Genital or perineal trauma	887	4 (0.5)	0.2 - 1.2	509	3 (0.6)	0.2 - 1.7
Mild or moderate vaginal bleeding	1'598	10 (0.6)	0.3 - 1.1	n. e.		
Heavy vaginal bleeding or PPH	6'429	1'750 (27.2)	26.1 - 28.3	3'311	3'226 (97.4)	96.8 - 97.9
Other intrapartum complications	3'189	73 (2.3)	1.8 - 2.9	6'711	958 (14.3)	13.5 - 15.1
Caesarean section	n. e.			n. e.		

Data is n (%) of observed women.

Of the women in the second trimester of pregnancy, 9'226 with the indication cervical ripening and/or labour induction and 14'613 with the indication abortion induction were observed for the events during delivery listed in table 28.

Table 28: Delivery outcome in the second trimester of pregnancy

Event	Cervical ripening and labour induction			Abortion induction		
	Total	With event	CI 95%	Total	With event	CI 95%
Hyperstimulation syndrome	232	66 (28.4)	23.0 - 34.6	n. e.		
Uterine dehiscence or rupture	n. e.			n. e.		
Genital or perineal trauma	6'661	5 (0.1)	0.0 -0.2	1'805	10 (0.6)	0.3 - 1.0
Mild or moderate vaginal bleeding	2'258	17 (0.8)	0.5 -1.2	n. e.		
Heavy vaginal bleeding or PPH	n. e.			609	306 (50.2)	46.3 - 54.2
Other intrapartum complications	8'838	10 (0.1)	0.1 - 0.2	8'210	390 (4.8)	4.3 - 5.2
Caesarean section	n. e.			n. e.		

Data is n (%) of observed women.

Of the women in the third trimester of pregnancy, 28'260 with the indication cervical ripening and/or labour induction were observed for the events during delivery listed in table 29.

Table 29: Delivery outcome in the third trimester of pregnancy

	Cervical ripening and labour induction		
Event	Total	With event	CI 95%
Hyperstimulation syndrome	19'961	3'050 (15.3)	14.8 - 15.8
Uterine dehiscence or rupture	18'638	1'271 (6.8)	6.5 - 7.2
Genital or perineal trauma	3'160	26 (0.8)	0.6 - 1.2
Mild or moderate vaginal bleeding	1'601	332 (20.7)	18.8 - 22.8
Heavy vaginal bleeding or PPH	1'108	43 (3.9)	2.9 - 5.2
Other intrapartum complications	10'307	739 (7.2)	6.7 - 7.7
Caesarean section	3'794	37 (1.0)	0.7 - 1.3

Data is n (%) of observed women.

4.4.3 Delivery Outcome by Indications

To assess whether the delivery outcome varies between the detailed indications, data was compared by regarding the different subgroups within the three main indications.

Of the women observed for the events during delivery listed in table 30, 23'197 received misoprostol only for cervical ripening, 7'166 only for labour induction, and 20'984 for both indications.

Table 30: Delivery outcome of women with indication cervical ripening and labour induction

Event	Only cervical ripening Total	With event	CI 95%	Only labour induction Total	With event	CI 95%	Cervical ripening and labour induction Total	With event	CI 95%
Hyperstimulation syndrome	578	86 (14.9)	12.2 - 18.0	4'437	291 (6.6)	5.9- 7.3	13'877	965 (7.0)	6.5 - 7.4
Uterine dehiscence or	8'197	12 (0.1)	0.1 - 0.3	2'130	9 (0.4)	0.2 - 0.8	976	15 (1.5)	0.9 - 2.5
Genital or perineal trauma	4'131	63 (1.5)	1.2 - 1.9	1'145	287 (25.1)	22.6 - 27.7	432	22 (5.1)	3.4 - 7.6
Mild or moderate vaginal bleeding	7'108	1'855 (26.1)	25.1 - 27.1	689	32 (4.6)	3.3 - 6.5	419	11 (2.6)	1.5 - 4.6
Heavy vaginal bleeding or PPH	13'055	93 (0.7)	0.6 - 0.9	5'181	470 (9.1)	8.3 - 9.9	5'365	285 (5.3)	4.7 - 5.9
Other intrapartum complications	50	2 (4.0)	1.1 - 13.5	1'431	20 (1.4)	0.9 - 2.1	2'548	43 (1.7)	1.3 - 2.3
Caesarean section	1026	235 (22.9)	20.4 - 25.6	6'608	1'166 (17.6)	16.7 - 18.6	19'903	4'566 (22.9)	22.4 - 23.5

Data is n (%) of observed women.

Of the women observed for the events during delivery listed in table 31, 20'365 received misoprostol for first-trimester abortions and 14'643 for second-trimester abortions.

Table 31: Delivery outcome of women with indication abortion induction

	First trimester abortion			Second trimester abortion		
Event	Total	With event	CI 95%	Total	With event	CI 95%
Hyperstimulation syndrome	n. e.			n. e.		
Uterine dehiscence or rupture	65	2 (3.1)	0.8 - 10.5	1'805	10 (0.6)	0.3 - 1.0
Genital or perineal trauma	n. e.			n. e.		
Mild or moderate vaginal bleeding	2'984	2'729 (91.5)	90.4 - 92.4	609	306 (50.2)	46.3 - 54.2
Heavy vaginal bleeding or PPH	6'384	947 (14.8)	14.0 - 15.7	8'210	390 (4.8)	4.3 - 5.2
Other intrapartum complications	n. e.			n. e.		
Caesarean section	n. e.			n. e.		

Data is n (%) of observed women.

Heavy vaginal bleeding occurred in 14.7% (CI 95%: 14.3-15.2) of the 25'183 observed women with the indication prevention of PPH. Other parameters were not evaluated for this indication. Treatment of PPH was not evaluated at all.

4.4.4 Delivery Outcome by different Modes of Application of Misoprostol

To evaluate whether the mode of application influences the outcome of delivery, data of women receiving misoprostol orally and vaginally was compared in all indications.

10'744 women with the indication cervical ripening and/or labour induction and 4'400 women with the indication abortion induction receiving misoprostol orally were observed for the events during delivery listed in table 32.

Table 32: Delivery outcome: oral application

	Cervical ripening and labour induction			Abortion induction		
Event	Total	With event	CI 95%	Total	With event	CI 95%
Hyperstimulation syndrome	4'529	854 (18.9)	17.7 - 20.0	n. e.		
Uterine dehiscence or rupture	4'514	388 (8.6)	7.8 - 9.4	n. e.		
Genital or perineal trauma	1'256	3 (0.2)	0.1 - 0.7	1*	1	
Mild or moderate vaginal bleeding	1'371	151 (11.0)	9.5 - 12.8	n. e.		
Heavy vaginal bleeding or PPH	4'865	749 (15.4)	14.4 - 16.4	1'475	1'261 (85.5)	83.6 - 87.2
Other intrapartum complications	3'969	292 (7.4)	6.6 - 8.2	1'724	403 (23.4)	21.4 - 25.4
Caesarean section	733	7 (1.0)	0.5 - 2.0	n. e.		

* Single case report

Data is n (%) of observed women.

25'356 women with the indication cervical ripening and/or labour induction and 24'228 women with the indication abortion induction receiving misoprostol vaginally were observed for the events during delivery listed in table 33.

Table 33: Delivery outcome: vaginal application

Event	Cervical ripening and labour induction			Abortion induction		
	Total	With event	CI 95%	Total	With event	CI 95%
Uterine contraction abnormalities without FHRch*	14'439	2'130 (14.8)	14.2 - 15.3	n. e.		
Hyperstimulation syndrome	12'988	820 (6.3)	5.9 - 6.7	n. e.		
Uterine dehiscence/rupture	3'426	29 (0.8)	0.6 - 1.2	1'619	9 (0.6)	0.3 - 1.1
Genital or perineal trauma	959	197 (20.5)	18.1 - 23.2	n. e.		
Mild or moderate vaginal bleeding	2'391	763 (31.9)	30.1 - 33.8	1'996	1'619 (81.1)	79.3 - 82.8
Heavy vaginal bleeding or PPH	9'331	461 (4.9)	4.5 - 5.4	12'081	937 (7.8)	7.3 - 8.2
Other intrapartum complications	2'862	52 (1.8)	1.4 - 2.4	n. e.		
Caesarean section	19'046	4'219 (22.2)	21.6 - 22.7	n. e.		

*Foetal heart-rate changes

Data is n (%) of observed women.

The frequency of uterine contraction anomalies with and without foetal heart-rate changes was almost similar between oral, vaginal, and sublingual application (14.8% CI 95%: 14.2-15.3, 18.9% CI 95%: 17.7-20.0 and 13.4% CI 95%: 10.9-17.3 without and 8.6% CI 95%:7.8-9.4, 6.3% CI 95%: 5.9-6.7, 6.5% CI 95%: 4.8-8.8 with FHRch respectively); rectal administration was not evaluated for this parameter.

4.4.5 Delivery Outcome by different Doses

To evaluate whether the outcome of delivery is influenced by the dose of the applied drug, the data was divided into a low and a high-dose group. As for the ADR the division was made according to the frequency of women of the used a specific dose..

Of the women with the indication cervical ripening and/or labour induction observed for the events during delivery listed in table 34, 4'608 received ≤ 300 µg and 6'136 received > 300 µg oral misoprostol per day.

Table 34: Delivery outcome: ≤ 300 µg vs. > 300 µg misoprostol administered orally

	≤ 300 µg/24 h			> 300 µg/24 h		
Event	Total	With event	CI 95%	Total	With event	CI 95%
Uterine contraction abnormalities without FHRch	1'986	452 (22.8)	21.0 - 24.7	2'543	402 (15.8)	14.4 - 17.3
Hyperstimulation syndrome	2'127	194 (9.1)	8.0 - 10.4	2'387	194 (8.1)	7.1 - 9.3
Uterine dehiscence/rupture	275	1 (0.4)	0.1 - 2.0	981	2 (0.2)	0.1 - 0.7
Genital or perineal trauma	634	123 (19.4)	16.5 - 22.7	737	28 (3.8)	2.6 - 5.4
Mild or moderate vaginal bleeding	1'391	164 (11.8)	10.2 - 13.6	3'474	585 (16.8)	15.6 - 18.1
Heavy vaginal bleeding or PPH	1'986	117 (5.9)	4.9 - 7.0	1'983	175 (8.8)	7.7 - 10.2
Other intrapartum complications	230	3 (1.3)	0.4 - 3.8	503	4 (0.8)	0.3 - 2.0
Caesarean section	3'469	700 (20.2)	18.9 - 21.5	3'057	592 (19.4)	18.0 - 20.8

Data is n (%) of observed women.

Of the women with the indication cervical ripening and/or labour induction observed for the events during delivery listed in table 35,

16'877 received ≤ 200 μg and 28'784 received > 200 μg vaginal misoprostol.

Table 35: Delivery outcome: ≤ 200 μg vs. > 200 μg misoprostol administered vaginally

	≤ 200 μg/24 h			> 200 μg/24 h		
Event	Total	With event	CI 95%	Total	With event	CI 95%
Uterine contraction abnormalities without FHRch	11'628	1'502 (12.9)	12.3 - 13.5	2'811	628 (22.3)	20.8 - 23.9
Hyperstimulation syndrome	10'188	531 (5.2)	4.8 - 5.7	2'800	289 (10.3)	9.2 - 11.5
Uterine dehiscence/rupture	2'804	16 (0.6)	0.4 - 0.9	622	13 (2.1)	1.2 - 3.5
Genital or perineal trauma	521	110 (21.1)	17.8 - 24.8	438	87 (19.9)	16.4 - 23.9
Mild or moderate vaginal bleeding	705	276 (39.1)	35.6 - 42.8	1'686	487 (28.9)	26.8 - 31.1
Heavy vaginal bleeding or PPH	7'679	401 (5.2)	4.7 - 5.7	1'652	60 (3.6)	2.8 - 4.6
Other intrapartum complications	2'043	36 (2.0)	1.3 - 2.4	819	16 (2.0)	1.2 - 3.1
Caesarean section	15'326	3'411 (22.3)	21.6 - 22.9	3'720	808 (21.7)	20.4 - 23.1

Data is n (%) of observed women.

4.4.6 Delivery Outcome with Misoprostol alone vs. in Combination with Oxytocin

To analyse whether the additional use of oxytocin influences the outcome of pregnancy, the data of women receiving misoprostol alone was compared to the data of women who received both misoprostol and oxytocin.

29'066 women with the indication cervical ripening and/or labour induction and 37'497 with the indication abortion induction received misoprostol alone and were observed for the events during delivery listed in table 36.

Table 36: Delivery outcome with misoprostol alone

	Cervical ripening and labour induction			Abortion induction		
Event	Total	With event	CI 95%	Total	With event	CI 95%
Hyperstimulation syndrome	18'984	2'952 (15.5)	15.0 - 16.1	n. e.		
Uterine dehiscence / rupture	18'154	1'269 (7.0)	6.6 - 7.4	n. e.		
Genital or perineal trauma	3'158	24 (0.8)	0.5 - 1.1	2'513	13 (0.5)	0.3 - 0.9
Mild or moderate vaginal bleeding	1'577	316 (20.0)	18.1 - 22.1	n. e.		
Heavy vaginal bleeding or PPH	940	34 (3.6)	2.6 - 5.0	4'520	3'642 (80.6)	79.4 - 81.7
Other intrapartum complications	10'517	711 (6.8)	6.3 - 7.3	16'128	1'542 (9.6)	9.1 - 10.0
Caesarean section	4'029	65 (1.6)	1.4 - 2.4	n. e.		

Data is n (%) of observed women.

882 women with the indication cervical ripening and/or labour induction and 1'742 with the indication abortion induction received misoprostol in combination with oxytocin and were observed for the events during delivery listed in table 37.

Table 37: Delivery outcome with misoprostol in combination with oxytocin

	Cervical ripening and labour induction			Abortion induction		
Event	Total	With event	CI 95%	Total	With event	CI 95%
Hyperstimulation syndrome	596	33 (5.5)	4.0 - 7.7	n. e.		
Uterine dehiscence / rupture	250	9 (3.6)	1.9 - 6.7	n. e.		
Genital or perineal trauma	2*	2		1*	1	
Mild or moderate vaginal bleeding	275	29 (10.5)	7.4 - 14.7	n. e.		
Heavy vaginal bleeding or PPH	n. e.			n. e.		
Other intrapartum complications	196	6 (3.1)	1.4 - 6.5	576	30 (5.2)	3.7 - 7.3
Caesarean section	n. e.			n. e.		

* Single case reports

Data is n (%) of observed women.

93'577 women receiving medication with misoprostol alone were compared to 7'122 women receiving misoprostol in combination with oxytocin for the events during delivery listed in table 38. Medication with misoprostol was given for all three main indications.

Table 38: Comparison of misoprostol alone vs. misoprostol in combination with oxytocin in all indications

	Misoprostol alone			Misoprostol with oxytocin		
Event	Total	With event	CI 95%	Total	With event	CI 95%
Uterine contraction abnormalities without FHRch	18'984	2'952 (15.5)	15.0 - 16.1	596	33 (5.5)	4.0 - 7.7
Hyperstimulation syndrome	18'154	1'269 (7.0)	6.6 - 7.4	250	9 (3.6)	1.9 - 6.7
Uterine dehiscence/rupture	5'671	37 (0.7)	0.5 - 0.9	3⁺	3	
Genital or perineal trauma	1'577	316 (20.0)	18.1 - 22.1	275	29 (10.5)	7.4 - 14.7
Mild or moderate vaginal bleeding	5'460	3'676 (67.3)	66.1 - 68.6	n. e.		
Heavy vaginal bleeding or PPH	49'970	6'123 (12.3)	12.0 - 12.5	4'274	411 (9.6)	8.8 - 10.5
Other intrapartum complications	2'502	46 (1.8)	1.4 - 2.4	n. e.		
Caesarean section	21'112	4'567 (21.6)	21.1 - 22.2	784	156 (19.9)	17.3 - 22.8

*Foetal heart-rate changes
⁺ Single case reports

Data is n (%) of observed women.

Regarding only data taken from RCTs, a total of 27'223 women with the indication cervical ripening and/or labour induction, 19'843 with abortion induction, and 29'117 with the prevention or treatment of PPH was observed for the events during birth listed in table 39.

Table 39: Delivery outcome only in RCTs

	Cervical ripening and labour induction			Abortion induction		
Event	Total	With event	CI 95%	Total	With event	CI 95%
Uterine contraction abnormalities without FHRch*	16'536	3'077 (18.6)	18.0 - 19.2	n. e.		
Hyperstimulation syndrome	15'483	1'253 (8.1)	7.7 - 8.5	n. e.		
Uterine dehiscence / rupture	1'375	12 (0.9)	0.5 - 1.5	64	1 (1.6)	0.3 - 8.3
Genital or perineal trauma	2'413	335 (13.9)	12.6 - 15.3	n. e.		
Mild or moderate vaginal bleeding	5'905	1'689 (28.6)	27.5 - 29.8	2'339	2'069 (88.5)	87.1 - 89.7
Heavy vaginal bleeding or PPH	8'155	555 (6.8)	6.3 - 7.4	5'887	711 (12.1)	11.3 - 12.9
Other intrapartum complications	2'413	45 (1.9)	1.4 - 2.5	n. e.		
Caesarean section	19'881	4'380 (22.0)	21.5 - 22.6	n. e.		

*Foetal heart-rate changes

Data is n (%) of observed women.

In the indication prevention of PPH heavy vaginal bleeding occurred in 15.4% (CI 95%: 15.0 - 15.9). Other parameters were not evaluated.

4.5 Neonatal Outcome

4.5.1 Overview

The data of newborns of women treated with misoprostol for cervical ripening and labour induction were evaluated.

A total of 27'350 newborns were observed for the ADR listed in table 40.

Table 40: Overview of neonatal ADR in all newborns

ADR	Total	With ADR	CI 95%
Apgar score ≤6 at 5 min	15'706	476 (3.0)	2.8 - 3.3
Admission to NICU	19'407	1'920 (9.9)	9.5 - 10.3
Presence of signs of foetal distress	19'082	3'629 (19.0)	18.5 - 19.6
Neonatal death	52'379	66 (0.1)	0.1 - 0.2
Other neonatal ADR	8'590	1'185 (13.8)	13.1 - 14.5

Data is n (%) of observed newborns.

4.5.2 Neonatal ADR by different Modes of Application of Misoprostol

10'744 newborns were observed for ADR after oral application of misoprostol and 25'356 after vaginal application.

Table 41: Neonatal ADR: oral vs. vaginal application

	Oral application			Vaginal application		
ADR	Total	With ADR	CI 95%	Total	With ADR	CI 95%
Apgar score ≤6 at 5 min	4'147	123 (3.0)	2.5 - 3.5	10'044	308 (3.1)	2.7 - 3.4
Admission to NICU	4'642	395 (8.5)	7.7 - 9.3	13'435	1'428 (10.6)	10.1 - 11.2
Presence of signs of foetal distress	4'906	829 (16.9)	15.9 - 18.0	12'640	2'363 (18.7)	18.0 - 19.4
Neonatal death	10'744	3 (0.0)	0.0 - 0.1	25'356	60 (0.2)	0.2 - 0.3
Other neonatal ADR	1'989	254 (12.8)	11.4 - 14.3	6'501	925 (14.2)	13.4 - 15.1

Data is n (%) of observed newborns.

4.5.3 Neonatal ADR by different Doses

4'362 newborns were observed for the ADR listed in table 43 after oral application of ≤300 µg misoprostol and 6'382 after oral application of >300 µg per day.

Table 42: Neonatal ADR: ≤ 300 µg vs. > 300 µg misoprostol administered orally

	≤ 300 µg/24 h			> 300 µg/24 h		
ADR	Total	With ADR	CI 95%	Total	With ADR	CI 95%
Apgar score ≤6 at 5 min	1'897	63 (3.3)	2.6 - 4.2	2'250	60 (2.7)	2.1 - 3.4
Admission to NICU	1'995	168 (8.4)	7.3 - 9.7	2'647	227 (8.6)	7.6 - 9.7
Presence of signs of foetal distress	2'238	322 (14.4)	13.0 - 15.9	2'668	507 (19.0)	17.6 - 20.5
Neonatal death	4'362	1 (0.0)	0.0 - 0.1	6'382	2 (0.0)	0.0 - 0.1
Other neonatal ADR	857	119 (13.9)	11.7 - 16.4	1'132	135 (11.9)	10.2 - 13.9

Data is n (%) of observed newborns.

16'877 newborns were observed for ADR after vaginal application of ≤200 µg misoprostol and 8'479 after vaginal application of >200 µg per day.

Table 43: Neonatal ADR: ≤ 200 µg vs. > 200 µg misoprostol administered vaginally

	≤ 200 µg/24 h			> 200 µg/24 h		
ADR	Total	With ADR	CI 95%	Total	With ADR	CI 95%
Apgar score ≤6 at 5 min	7'413	223 (3.0)	2.6 - 3.4	2'631	85 (3.2)	2.6 –4.0
Admission to NICU	10'928	1'206 (11.0)	10.5 - 11.6	2'507	222 (8.9)	7.8 - 10.0
Presence of signs of foetal distress	9'567	1'754 (18.3)	17.6 - 19.1	3'073	609 (19.8)	18.4 - 21.3
Neonatal death	16'877	59 (0.3)	0.3 - 0.5	8'479	1 (0.0)	0.0 - 0.1
Other neonatal ADR	5'978	883 (14.8)	13.9 - 15.7	523	42 (8.0)	6.0 - 10.7

Data is n (%) of observed newborns.

4.6 Performed Meta-analyses of Maternal Adverse Drug Reactions and Delivery

In a second step of analysis, only the data of RCT was collected and evaluated. The data of RCT comparing the same treatment regimens was scheduled and analysed by meta-analysis.

In order to compare the frequency of ADR in women receiving misoprostol administered with different modes and other drugs instead of misoprostol for the three obstetrical indications, 35 meta-analyses were conducted. The parameters gastrointestinal ADR, fever and shivering as maternal ADR and the uterine hyperstimulation syndrome (= uterine contraction abnormalities with foetal heart-rate changes) and caesarean section as indicators for outcome of delivery were evaluated.

4.6.1 GIT Disturbances

Table 44: Meta-analyses performed for GIT disturbances

Comparison	Recruited studies (N)	Studies used (N)	RR random	CI 95%
Indication: Cervical ripening and labour induction				
Different mode of application				
Oral vs. vaginal misoprostol	31	17	1.90	1.17 – 3.09
Sublingual vs. vaginal misoprostol	9	6	1.67	0.95 – 2.96
Oral vs. sublingual misoprostol	4	2	0.49	0.08 – 3.06

Misoprostol vs. other uterotonics				
Oral misoprostol vs. vaginal or cervical PGE2	12	7	1.21	0.82 – 1.79
Vaginal misoprostol vs. IMN	7	4	1.73	0.70 – 4.30
Indication: Abortion induction				
Different mode of application				
Oral vs. vaginal misoprostol	12	7	1.42	0.97 – 2.08
Sublingual vs. vaginal misoprostol	9	8	1.24	1.02 – 1.51
Oral vs. sublingual misoprostol	4	4	1.45	0.73 – 2.87
Different doses				
400 vs. 600 µg vaginal misoprostol	5	5	0.91	0.68 – 1.23
Misoprostol vs. placebo				
Vaginal misoprostol vs. placebo	4	3	1.12	0.86 – 1.45
Misoprostol vs. other uterotonics				
Vaginal misoprostol vs. vaginal gemeprost	4	4	0.59	0.44 – 0.79

Prevention of PPH				
Misoprostol vs. placebo				
Oral misoprostol vs. placebo	6	3	2.94	0.84–10.23
Misoprostol vs. other uterotonics				
Oral misoprostol vs. i.m. oxytocin	12	11	1.51	0.89 – 2.56

N = number of studies

Figures 4 and 5 illustrate the incidence of gastrointestinal ADR when oral misoprostol was compared to vaginal misoprostol and vaginal or cervical PGE2 for cervical ripening and labour induction. Table 45 shows the comparison of vaginal misoprostol to oxytocin, when used for the prevention of PPH.

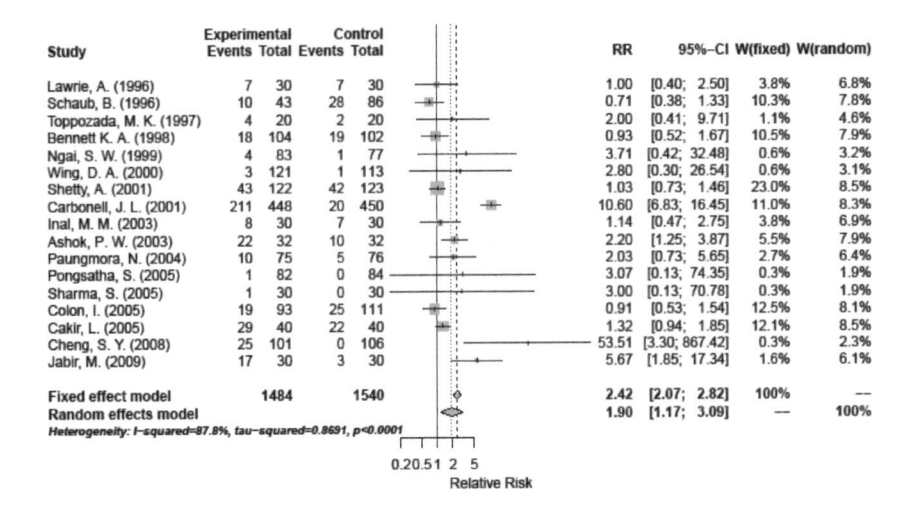

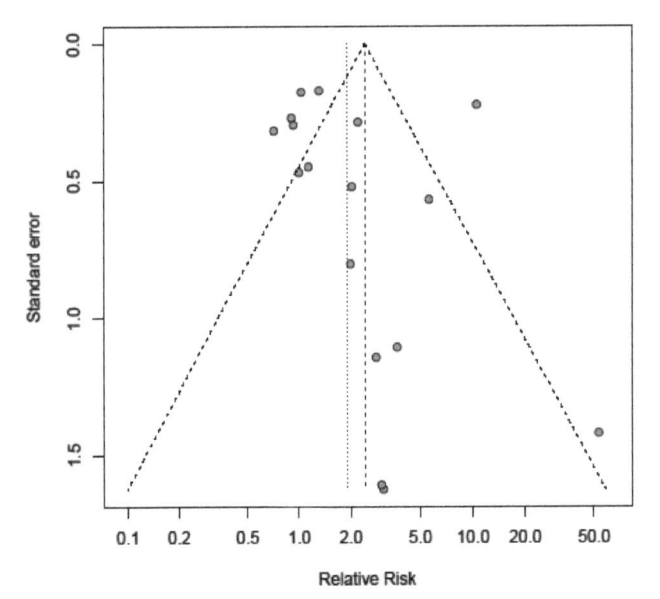

Study	Experimental Events Total	Control Events Total	RR	95%-CI	W(fixed)	W(random)
Lawrie, A. (1996)	7 30	7 30	1.00	[0.40; 2.50]	3.8%	6.8%
Schaub, B. (1996)	10 43	28 86	0.71	[0.38; 1.33]	10.3%	7.8%
Toppozada, M. K. (1997)	4 20	2 20	2.00	[0.41; 9.71]	1.1%	4.6%
Bennett K. A. (1998)	18 104	19 102	0.93	[0.52; 1.67]	10.5%	7.9%
Ngai, S. W. (1999)	4 83	1 77	3.71	[0.42; 32.48]	0.6%	3.2%
Wing, D. A. (2000)	3 121	1 113	2.80	[0.30; 26.54]	0.6%	3.1%
Shetty, A. (2001)	43 122	42 123	1.03	[0.73; 1.46]	23.0%	8.5%
Carbonell, J. L. (2001)	211 448	20 450	10.60	[6.83; 16.45]	11.0%	8.3%
Inal, M. M. (2003)	8 30	7 30	1.14	[0.47; 2.75]	3.8%	6.9%
Ashok, P. W. (2003)	22 32	10 32	2.20	[1.25; 3.87]	5.5%	7.9%
Paungmora, N. (2004)	10 75	5 76	2.03	[0.73; 5.65]	2.7%	6.4%
Pongsatha, S. (2005)	1 82	0 84	3.07	[0.13; 74.35]	0.3%	1.9%
Sharma, S. (2005)	1 30	0 30	3.00	[0.13; 70.78]	0.3%	1.9%
Colon, I. (2005)	19 93	25 111	0.91	[0.53; 1.54]	12.5%	8.1%
Cakir, L. (2005)	29 40	22 40	1.32	[0.94; 1.85]	12.1%	8.5%
Cheng, S. Y. (2008)	25 101	0 106	53.51	[3.30; 867.42]	0.3%	2.3%
Jabir, M. (2009)	17 30	3 30	5.67	[1.85; 17.34]	1.6%	6.1%
Fixed effect model	1484	1540	2.42	[2.07; 2.82]	100%	—
Random effects model			1.90	[1.17; 3.09]	—	100%

Heterogeneity: I-squared=87.8%, tau-squared=0.8691, p<0.0001

Figure 4: Gastrointestinal ADR with oral vs. vaginal misoprostol for cervical ripening and labour induction (Experimental = oral misoprostol, control = vaginal misoprostol)

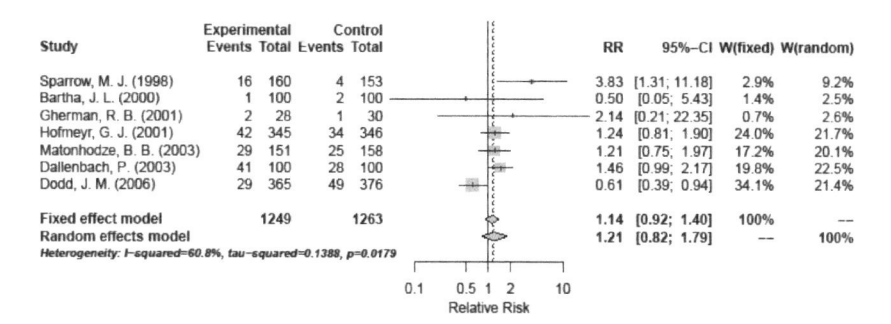

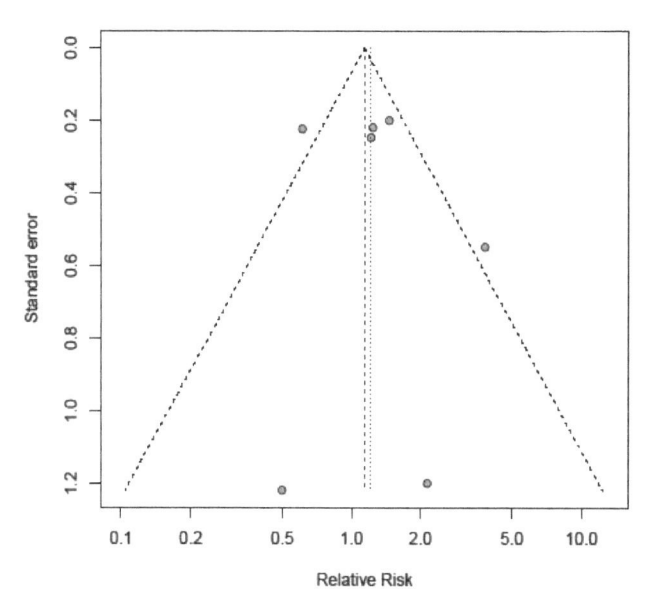

Study	Experimental Events	Total	Control Events	Total	RR	95%-CI	W(fixed)	W(random)
Sparrow, M. J. (1998)	16	160	4	153	3.83	[1.31; 11.18]	2.9%	9.2%
Bartha, J. L. (2000)	1	100	2	100	0.50	[0.05; 5.43]	1.4%	2.5%
Gherman, R. B. (2001)	2	28	1	30	2.14	[0.21; 22.35]	0.7%	2.6%
Hofmeyr, G. J. (2001)	42	345	34	346	1.24	[0.81; 1.90]	24.0%	21.7%
Matonhodze, B. B. (2003)	29	151	25	158	1.21	[0.75; 1.97]	17.2%	20.1%
Dallenbach, P. (2003)	41	100	28	100	1.46	[0.99; 2.17]	19.8%	22.5%
Dodd, J. M. (2006)	29	365	49	376	0.61	[0.39; 0.94]	34.1%	21.4%
Fixed effect model		1249		1263	1.14	[0.92; 1.40]	100%	--
Random effects model					1.21	[0.82; 1.79]	--	100%

Heterogeneity: I-squared=60.8%, tau-squared=0.1388, p=0.0179

Figure 5: Gastrointestinal ADR with oral misoprostol vs. vaginal or cervical PGE2 for cervical ripening and labour induction (Experimental = oral misoprostol, control = vaginal or cervical PGE2)

4.6.2 Fever and Shivering

Table 45: Meta-analyses performed for fever and shivering

Comparison	Recruited studies (N)	Studies used (N)	RR random	CI 95%
Cervical ripening and labour induction				
Different mode of application				
Oral vs. vaginal misoprostol	31	4	1.06	0.32 – 3.64
Sublingual vs. vaginal misoprostol	9	6	2.00	0.82 – 4.90
Oral vs. sublingual misoprostol	4	3	0.84	0.62 – 1.15
Abortion induction				
Different mode of application				
Oral vs. vaginal misoprostol	12	7	0.98	0.57 – 1.70
Sublingual vs. vaginal misoprostol	9	8	1.22	0.91 – 1.62
Oral vs. sublingual misoprostol	4	3	0.46	0.20 – 1.06
Different doses				
400 vs. 600 µg vaginal misoprostol	5	4	1.16	1.07 – 1.25
Misoprostol vs. other uterotonics				
Vaginal misoprostol vs. vaginal gemeprost	4	4	1.16	0.47 – 2.87

Prevention of PPH				
Misoprostol vs. placebo				
Oral misoprostol vs. placebo	6	6	8.09	3.54 – 18.46
Misoprostol vs. other uterotonics				
Oral misoprostol vs. i. m. oxytocin	12	11	3.17	2.05 – 4.90

N = number of studies

Figure 5 and 6 illustrate the incidence of fever and shivering after the application of misoprostol, comparing its use in the indications cervical ripening and labour induction and abortion induction when oral and vaginal application were compared. Figure 7 shows the incidence after the application of oral misoprostol compared to oxytocin when used for the prevention of PPH.

Study	Experimental Events Total	Control Events Total	RR	95%-CI	W(fixed)	W(random)
Schaub, B. (1996)	0 43	1 86	0.66	[0.03; 15.94]	1.5%	10.6%
Carbonell, J. L. (2001)	129 448	42 450	3.09	[2.23; 4.26]	61.9%	37.5%
Colon, I. (2005)	14 93	24 111	0.70	[0.38; 1.27]	32.3%	35.2%
Cheng, S. Y. (2008)	1 101	3 106	0.35	[0.04; 3.31]	4.3%	16.6%
Fixed effect model	685	753	2.16	[1.65; 2.82]	100%	--
Random effects model			1.08	[0.32; 3.64]	--	100%

Heterogeneity: I-squared=86%, tau-squared=1.001, p<0.0001

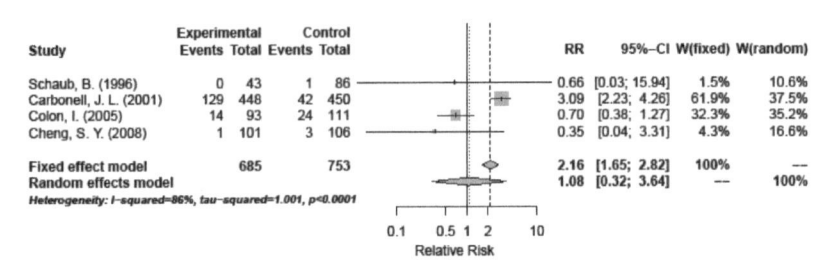

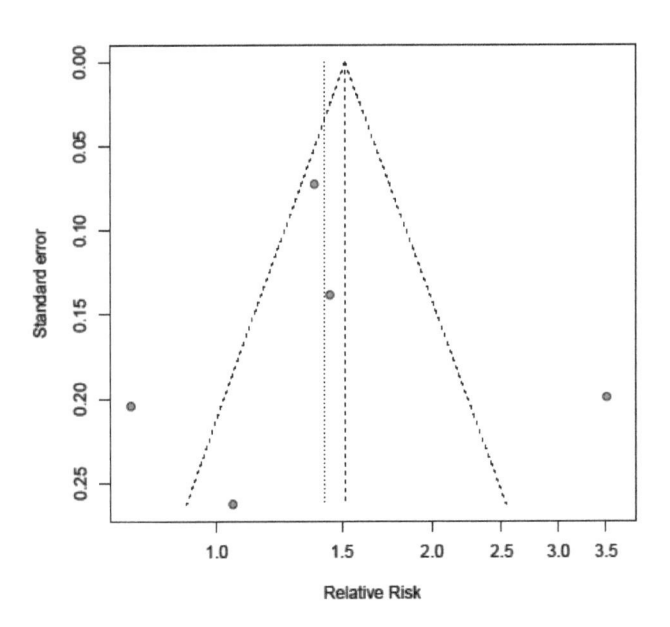

Figure 5: Fever / shivering with oral vs. vaginal misoprostol for cervical ripening and labour induction
(Experimental = oral misoprostol, control = vaginal misoprostol)

Study	Experimental Events Total	Control Events Total	RR	95%-CI	W(fixed)	W(random)
Creinin, M. D. (1997)	12 12	8 8			0.0%	0.0%
Pang, M. W. (2001)	80 103	21 95	3.51	[2.38; 5.20]	15.4%	19.3%
Ngoc, N. T. (2004)	28 95	37 95	0.76	[0.51; 1.13]	26.1%	19.1%
Akoury, H. A. (2004)	38 38	51 70	1.37	[1.19; 1.58]	25.4%	23.3%
Caliskan, E. (2005)	19 51	18 51	1.06	[0.63; 1.77]	12.7%	16.8%
Blanchard, K. (2005)	52 60	24 40	1.44	[1.10; 1.90]	20.3%	21.5%
Behrashi, M. (2008)	0 30	0 30			0.0%	0.0%
Fixed effect model	389	389	1.52	[1.31; 1.75]	100%	--
Random effects model			1.42	[0.97; 2.08]	--	100%

Heterogeneity: I-squared=87.9%, tau-squared=0.1682, p<0.0001

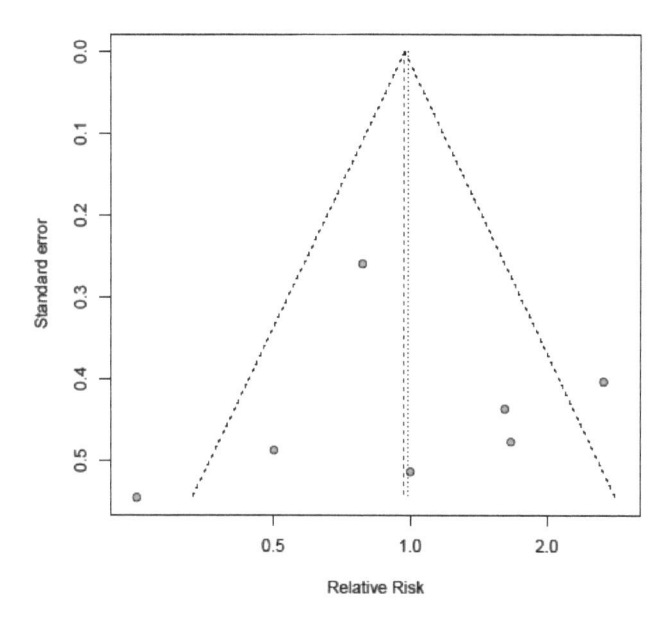

Figure 6: Fever / shivering with oral vs. vaginal misoprostol for abortion induction

(Experimental = oral misoprostol, control = vaginal misoprostol)

Study	Experimental Events Total	Control Events Total	RR	95%–CI	W(fixed)	W(random)
Cook, C. M. (1999)	136 424	68 439	2.07	[1.60; 2.68]	6.0%	12.7%
Walley, R. L. (2000)	51 154	15 164	3.62	[2.13; 6.16]	1.3%	11.1%
Acharya, G. (2001)	2 30	2 30	1.00	[0.15; 6.64]	0.2%	3.8%
Benchimol, M. (2001)	11 186	0 196	24.23	[1.44; 408.32]	0.0%	2.0%
Kundodyiwa, T. W. (2001)	124 243	79 256	1.65	[1.33; 2.06]	7.0%	12.8%
Gulmezoglu, A. M. (2001)	2179 9227	558 3232	1.37	[1.26; 1.49]	74.8%	13.2%
Lumbiganon, P. (2002)	294 843	60 843	4.90	[3.78; 6.36]	5.4%	12.7%
Oboro, V. O. (2003)	144 247	36 249	4.03	[2.93; 5.55]	3.2%	12.4%
Zachariah, E. S. (2006)	116 730	17 617	5.77	[3.51; 9.49]	1.7%	11.3%
Baskett, T. F. (2007)	60 311	1 311	60.00	[8.37; 430.23]	0.1%	3.6%
Afolabi, E. O. (2010)	4 100	2 100	2.00	[0.37; 10.67]	0.2%	4.5%
Fixed effect model	12495	6437	1.88	[1.75; 2.01]	100%	--
Random effects model			3.17	[2.05; 4.90]	--	100%

Heterogeneity: I-squared=94.2%, tau-squared=0.3813, p<0.0001

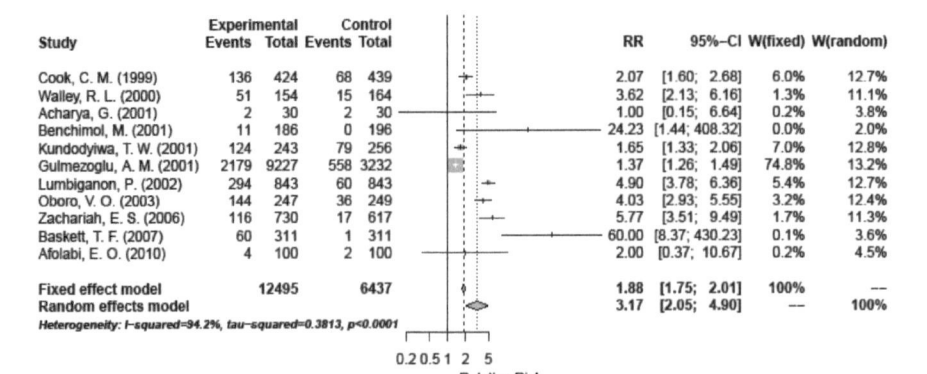

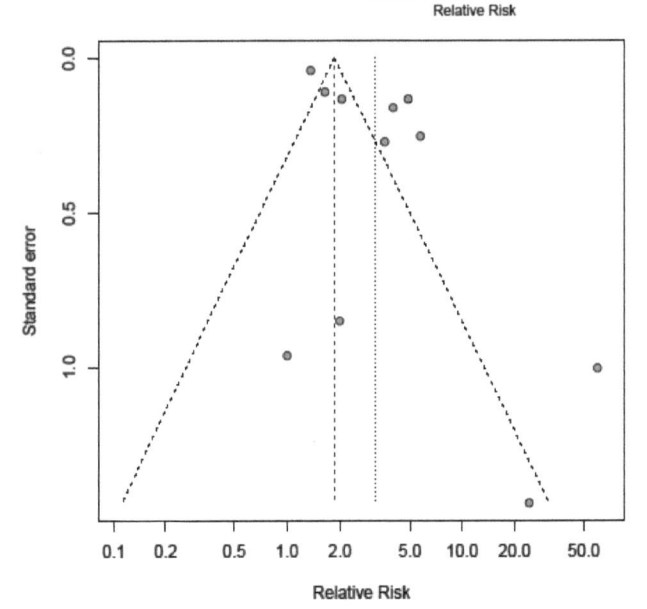

Figure 7: Fever / shivering with oral misoprostol vs. oxytocin for the prevention of PPH

(Experimental = oral misoprostol, control = oxytocin)

4.6.3 Hyperstimulation Syndrome (Uterine Contraction Abnormalities with Foetal Heart-Rate Changes)

Table 46: Meta-analyses performed for hyperstimulation syndrome

Comparison	Recruited studies (N)	Studies used (N)	RR random	CI 95%
Cervical ripening and labour induction				
Different doses				
25 vs. 50 µg vaginal misoprostol	8	6	0.61	0.31 – 1.21
Misoprostol vs. placebo				
Oral misoprostol vs. placebo	7	4	2.22	0.83 – 5.96
Vaginal misoprostol vs. placebo	13	2	1.93	0.42 – 8.95
Misoprostol vs. other uterotonics				
Oral misoprostol vs. vaginal or cervical PGE2	12	7	0.96	0.62 – 1.49
Vaginal misoprostol vs. vaginal or cervical PGE2	35	27	1.31	0.94 – 1.83
Vaginal misoprostol vs. oxytocin	12	6	1.06	0.49 – 2.28

N = number of studies

Figures 8 and 9 show the comparison of vaginal misoprostol to oxytocin and PGE2 for cervical ripening and labour induction concerning the incidence of hyperstimulation syndrome.

Study	Experimental Events Total	Control Events Total	RR	95%-CI	W(fixed)	W(random)
Sanchez-Ramos, L. (1993)	7 64	3 65	2.37	[0.64; 8.76]	8.4%	19.7%
Escudero, F. (1997)	5 57	0 63	12.15	[0.69; 214.89]	1.3%	6.2%
de Aquino, M. M. (2003)	3 105	4 105	0.75	[0.17; 3.27]	11.3%	17.1%
Zeteroglu, S. (2005)	1 48	2 49	0.51	[0.05; 5.45]	5.6%	8.6%
Gelisen, O. (2005)	3 100	2 100	1.50	[0.26; 8.79]	5.6%	13.4%
Fonseca, L. (2008)	13 164	24 163	0.54	[0.28; 1.02]	67.8%	34.9%
Fixed effect model	538	545	0.92	[0.59; 1.46]	100%	---
Random effects model			1.06	[0.49; 2.28]	---	100%

Heterogeneity: I-squared=40.7%, tau-squared=0.3593, p=0.134

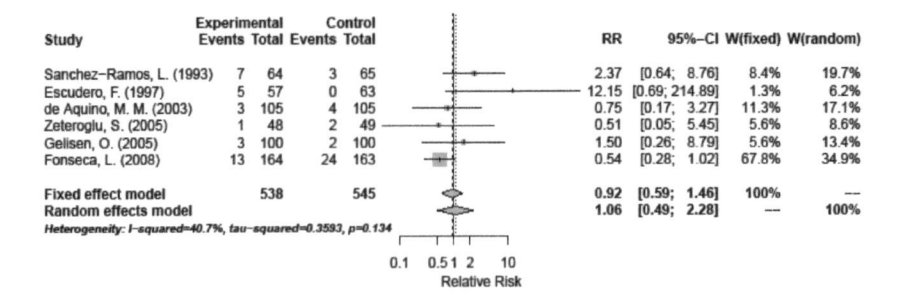

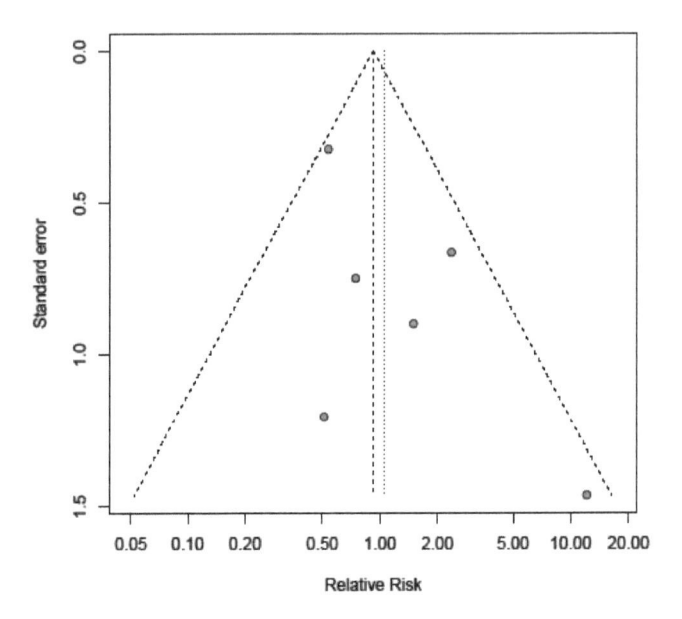

Figure 8: Hyperstimulation syndrome with vaginal misoprostol vs. oxytocin for cervical ripening and labour induction (Experimental = vaginal misoprostol, control = oxytocin)

Study	Experimental Events Total	Control Events Total		RR	95%-CI	W(fixed)	W(random)
Wing, D. A. (1995)	5 68	2 67		2.46	[0.49; 12.26]	1.9%	3.6%
Wing, D. A. (1995)	8 638	3 137		0.57	[0.15; 2.13]	4.6%	5.0%
Gottschall, D. S. (1997)	0 38	0 37				0.0%	0.0%
Herabutya, Y. (1997)	1 60	0 50		2.50	[0.10; 60.14]	0.5%	1.1%
Wing, D. A. (1997)	1 99	4 98		0.25	[0.03; 2.17]	3.8%	2.1%
Chang, C. H. (1997)	4 30	3 30		1.33	[0.33; 5.45]	2.8%	4.5%
Sanchez-Ramos, L. (1998)	12 108	9 115		1.42	[0.62; 3.23]	8.1%	9.2%
Nunes, F. (1999)	3 95	4 94		0.74	[0.17; 3.23]	3.8%	4.2%
Charoenkul, S. (2000)	5 72	0 71		10.85	[0.61; 192.59]	0.5%	1.3%
Khoury, A. N. (2001)	3 79	1 39		1.48	[0.16; 13.78]	1.3%	2.0%
Neiger, R. (2001)	4 32	0 29		8.17	[0.46; 145.37]	0.5%	1.3%
Rowlands, S. (2001)	10 63	0 63		21.00	[1.26; 350.78]	0.5%	1.3%
Frohn, W. E. (2002)	5 54	0 55		11.20	[0.63; 197.73]	0.5%	1.3%
Ayad, I. A. (2002)	5 118	1 120		5.08	[0.60; 42.87]	0.9%	2.2%
Urban, R. (2003)	1 44	0 40		2.73	[0.11; 65.14]	0.5%	1.1%
Garry, D. (2003)	4 97	1 89		3.67	[0.42; 32.22]	1.0%	2.1%
Ramsey, P. S. (2003)	5 38	3 73		3.20	[0.81; 12.68]	1.9%	4.6%
Lokugamage, A. U. (2003)	10 96	12 95		0.82	[0.37; 1.82]	11.3%	9.7%
Bolnick, J. M. (2004)	0 77	0 74				0.0%	0.0%
Sharma, Y. (2005)	2 23	1 21		1.83	[0.18; 18.70]	1.0%	1.9%
Ramsey, P. S. (2005)	5 38	4 73		2.40	[0.68; 8.42]	2.6%	5.3%
Denguezli, W. (2007)	5 65	3 65		1.67	[0.42; 6.69]	2.8%	4.5%
Krithika, K. S. (2008)	3 50	2 50		1.50	[0.26; 8.60]	1.9%	3.1%
Calder, A. A. (2008)	19 318	20 308		0.92	[0.50; 1.69]	19.0%	12.4%
Wing, D. A. (2008)	23 871	21 436		0.55	[0.31; 0.98]	26.1%	12.9%
Shakya, R. (2010)	0 35	0 31				0.0%	0.0%
Tan, T. C. (2010)	4 112	2 57		1.02	[0.19; 5.39]	2.5%	3.4%
Fixed effect model	3418	2417		1.28	[1.01; 1.63]	100%	--
Random effects model				1.31	[0.94; 1.83]	--	100%

Heterogeneity: I-squared=25.9%, tau-squared=0.1588, p=0.1217

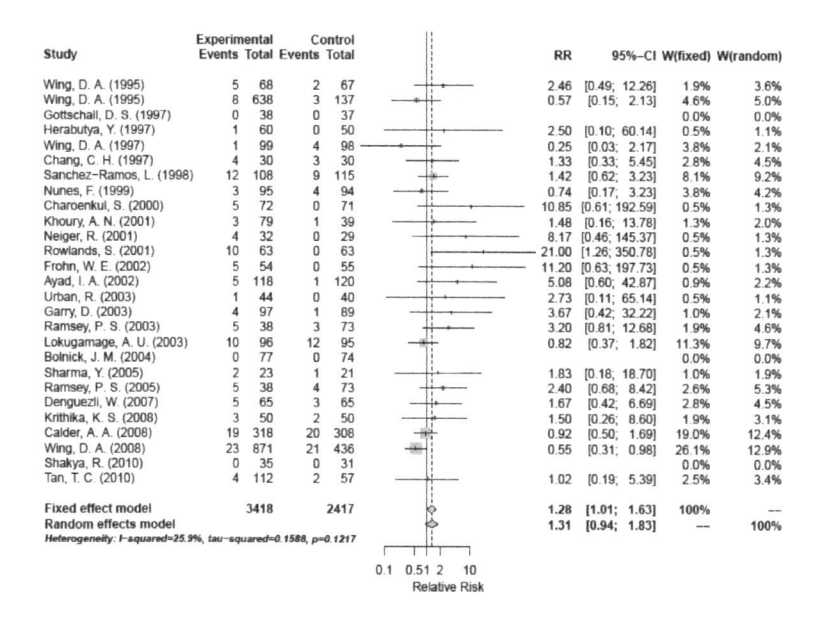

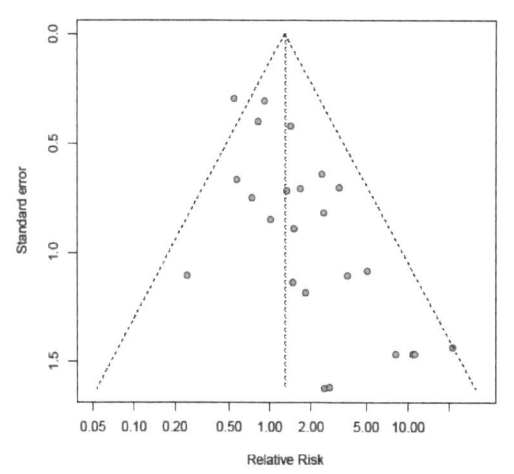

Figure 9: Hyperstimulation syndrome with vaginal misoprostol vs. PGE2 for cervical ripening and labour induction
(Experimental = vaginal misoprostol, control = vaginal or cervical PGE2)

4.6.4 Caesarean Section (CS)

Table 47: Meta-analyses performed for caesarean section

Comparison	Recruited studies (N)	Studies used (N)	RR random	CI 95%
Cervical ripening and labour induction				
Misoprostol vs. placebo				
Oral misoprostol vs. placebo	7	6	0.61	0.42 – 0.89
Vaginal misoprostol vs. placebo	13	3	1.09	0.68 – 1.74
Misoprostol vs. other uterotonics				
Oral misoprostol vs. vaginal or cervical PGE2	12	11	0.84	0.74 – 0.96
Oral misoprostol vs. oxytocin	6	4	0.95	0.66 – 1.35
Vaginal misoprostol vs. vaginal or cervical PGE2	35	33	0.97	0.85 – 1.10
Vaginal misoprostol vs. oxytocin	12	9	0.98	0.70 – 1.38

N = number of studies

The following figures 9-12 illustrate the comparison of misoprostol and placebo or other uterotonics (PGE2, oxytocin) concerning the rate of CS as a measure for efficacy.

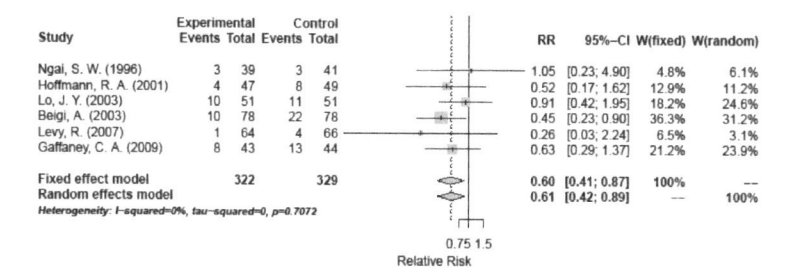

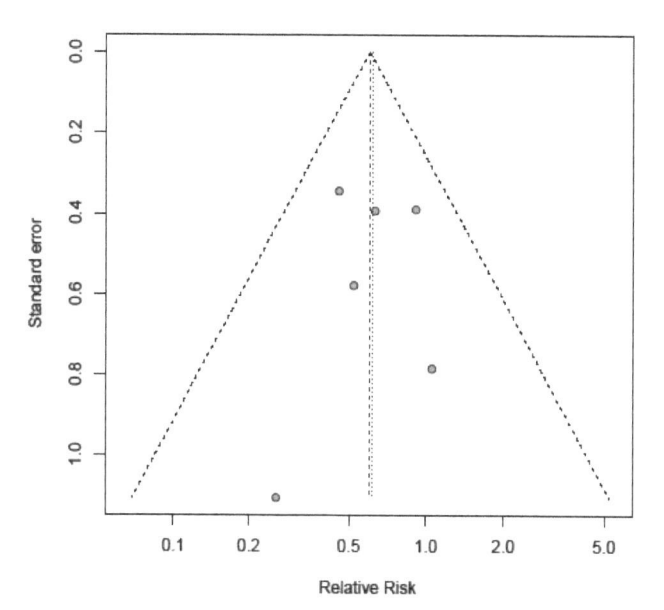

Study	Experimental Events	Total	Control Events	Total	RR	95%-CI	W(fixed)	W(random)
Ngai, S. W. (1996)	3	39	3	41	1.05	[0.23; 4.90]	4.8%	6.1%
Hoffmann, R. A. (2001)	4	47	8	49	0.52	[0.17; 1.62]	12.9%	11.2%
Lo, J. Y. (2003)	10	51	11	51	0.91	[0.42; 1.95]	18.2%	24.6%
Beigi, A. (2003)	10	78	22	78	0.45	[0.23; 0.90]	36.3%	31.2%
Levy, R. (2007)	1	64	4	66	0.26	[0.03; 2.24]	6.5%	3.1%
Gaffaney, C. A. (2009)	8	43	13	44	0.63	[0.29; 1.37]	21.2%	23.9%
Fixed effect model		322		329	0.60	[0.41; 0.87]	100%	---
Random effects model					0.61	[0.42; 0.89]	---	100%

Heterogeneity: I-squared=0%, tau-squared=0, p=0.7072

Figure 10: Caesarean section with oral misoprostol vs. placebo for cervical ripening and labour induction

(Experimental = oral misoprostol, control = placebo)

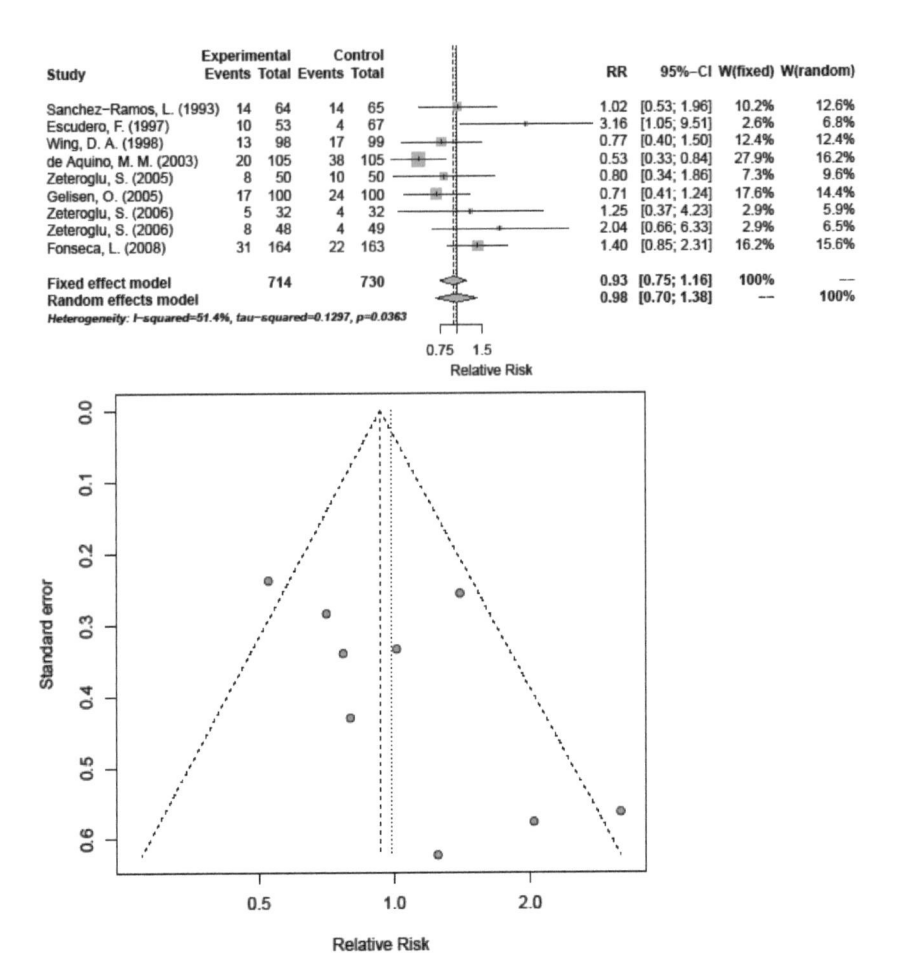

Study	Experimental Events	Total	Control Events	Total	RR	95%-CI	W(fixed)	W(random)
Sanchez-Ramos, L. (1993)	14	64	14	65	1.02	[0.53; 1.96]	10.2%	12.6%
Escudero, F. (1997)	10	53	4	67	3.16	[1.05; 9.51]	2.6%	6.8%
Wing, D. A. (1998)	13	98	17	99	0.77	[0.40; 1.50]	12.4%	12.4%
de Aquino, M. M. (2003)	20	105	38	105	0.53	[0.33; 0.84]	27.9%	16.2%
Zeteroglu, S. (2005)	8	50	10	50	0.80	[0.34; 1.86]	7.3%	9.6%
Gelisen, O. (2005)	17	100	24	100	0.71	[0.41; 1.24]	17.6%	14.4%
Zeteroglu, S. (2006)	5	32	4	32	1.25	[0.37; 4.23]	2.9%	5.9%
Zeteroglu, S. (2006)	8	48	4	49	2.04	[0.66; 6.33]	2.9%	6.5%
Fonseca, L. (2008)	31	164	22	163	1.40	[0.85; 2.31]	16.2%	15.6%
Fixed effect model		714		730	0.93	[0.75; 1.16]	100%	--
Random effects model					0.98	[0.70; 1.38]	--	100%

Heterogeneity: I-squared=51.4%, tau-squared=0.1297, p=0.0363

Figure 11: Caesarean section (CS) with vaginal misoprostol vs. oxytocin for cervical ripening and labour induction
(Experimental = vaginal misoprostol, control = oxytocin)

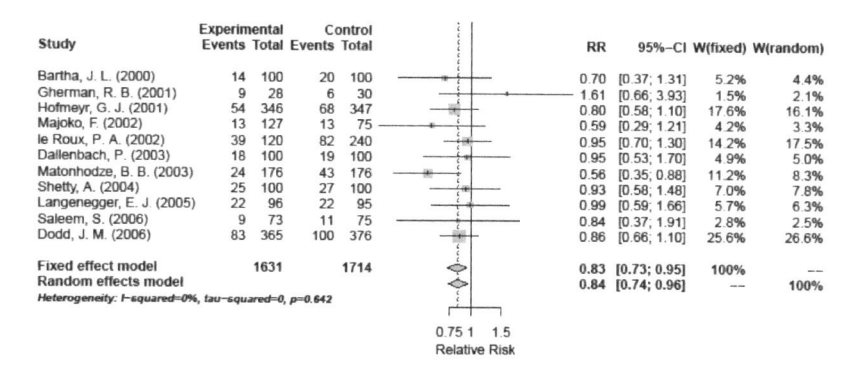

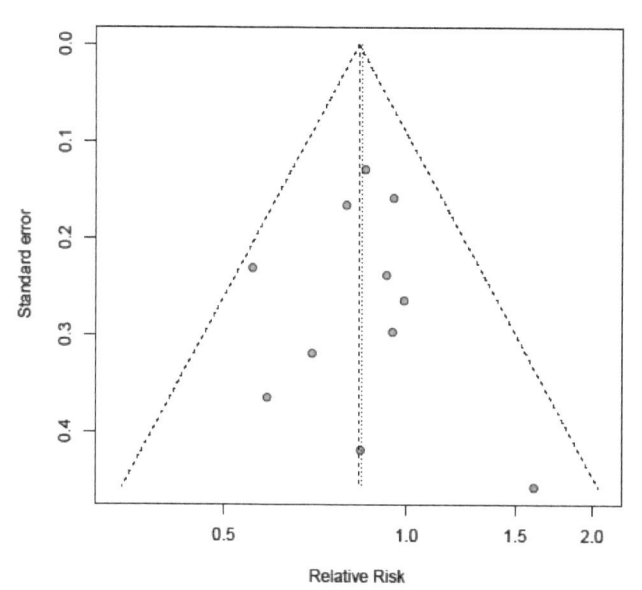

Study	Experimental Events Total	Control Events Total	RR	95%-CI	W(fixed)	W(random)
Bartha, J. L. (2000)	14 100	20 100	0.70	[0.37; 1.31]	5.2%	4.4%
Gherman, R. B. (2001)	9 28	6 30	1.61	[0.66; 3.93]	1.5%	2.1%
Hofmeyr, G. J. (2001)	54 346	68 347	0.80	[0.58; 1.10]	17.6%	16.1%
Majoko, F. (2002)	13 127	13 75	0.59	[0.29; 1.21]	4.2%	3.3%
le Roux, P. A. (2002)	39 120	82 240	0.95	[0.70; 1.30]	14.2%	17.5%
Dallenbach, P. (2003)	18 100	19 100	0.95	[0.53; 1.70]	4.9%	5.0%
Matonhodze, B. B. (2003)	24 176	43 176	0.56	[0.35; 0.88]	11.2%	8.3%
Shetty, A. (2004)	25 100	27 100	0.93	[0.58; 1.48]	7.0%	7.8%
Langenegger, E. J. (2005)	22 96	22 95	0.99	[0.59; 1.66]	5.7%	6.3%
Saleem, S. (2006)	9 73	11 75	0.84	[0.37; 1.91]	2.8%	2.5%
Dodd, J. M. (2006)	83 365	100 376	0.86	[0.66; 1.10]	25.6%	26.6%
Fixed effect model	1631	1714	0.83	[0.73; 0.95]	100%	--
Random effects model			0.84	[0.74; 0.96]	--	100%

Heterogeneity: I-squared=0%, tau-squared=0, p=0.642

Figure 12: Caesarean section (CS) with oral misoprostol vs. PGE2 for cervical ripening and labour induction (Experimental = oral misoprostol, control = vaginal or cervical PGE2)

5. Discussion

By pooling and evaluating data from studies published on the online database PubMed from 1987 until 2011 and investigating the use of misoprostol in its main obstetrical indications (cervical ripening and labour induction, abortion induction and prevention and treatment of PPH), an overview of the available information on the efficacy and safety of misoprostol in obstetrics was provided. The results of searches in PubMed including the key word "misoprostol", show that intensive research has already been conducted over the last 30 years and is still going on. This illustrates that the discussion on the use of misoprostol in obstetrics still arouses great interest.

5.1 Maternal Adverse Drug Reactions (ADR)

After medication with misoprostol, the most frequently observed maternal ADR were gastrointestinal ADR (including nausea, vomiting, and diarrhoea), fever and shivering. According to current literature, these ADR are dependent on the dose as well as on the mode of application of misoprostol [18].

In our study, these ADR were most frequently observed in women treated with misoprostol for the induction of abortion. Gastrointestinal ADR were present in up to 53.4% after first-trimester abortions and 34.6% after second-trimester abortions. Fever and shivering occurred in 38.1% after first and in 42.7% after second-trimester abortions. Regarding the fact, that doses used for the induction of abortion are usually many times higher than doses used for the two indications and, moreover, doses given for second-trimester abortions are higher than for first-trimester abortions, our results confirm this hypothesis.

However, we could not find any relevant dose dependence of gastrointestinal ADR. For vaginal application, gastrointestinal ADR were slightly more frequent after misoprostol doses of >200 µg per day than after ≤200 µg per day, however, after oral application, they were more frequent in case of ≤300 µg per day than >300 µg per day

The comparison of 400 vs. 600 µg per day of vaginally administered misoprostol for abortion induction showed a slight reduction of gastrointestinal ADR with a lower-dose regimen, but this is not statistically significant (RR random = 0.91, CI 95%: 0.68-1.23). Dodd et al. compared cumulative doses of <800 vs. 800-2400 vaginally administered misoprostol for termination of pregnancy in the second or third trimester and found no significant difference between the groups concerning the rate of gastrointestinal ADR (nausea: RR = 0.97, CI 95%: 0.59-1.59, vomiting RR = 0.58, CI 95%: 0.28-1.17, diarrhoea: RR = 2.26, 6.39, CI 95%: 0.80-6.39) [23].

Shivering and fever occurred more frequently in women receiving misoprostol for the induction of abortion (up to 42.7%, in the group with second-trimester abortions) and for the prevention of PPH, compared to the women needing cervical ripening and labour induction. When 400 vs. 600 µg vaginal misoprostol were compared, there was a significantly higher incidence of fever and shivering after application of the higher dose regimen (RR random = 1.16, CI 95%: 1.07-1.25).

In our study, the additional use of oxytocin does not result in an increase of the rate of any ADR. However, women treated with both drugs in combination suffered less frequently from gastrointestinal ADR. One reason could be that the he dose of misoprostol is usually lower when it is combined with oxytocin than when it is given alone.

Pharmacokinetic studies confirm that peak plasma concentration is reached faster after oral than after vaginal application. A pharmacokinetic study conducted by Khan et al., comparing plasma concentrations of 400 µg misoprostol administered orally, vaginally, or rectally before surgical termination of pregnancy in the first or second trimester, showed that after oral misoprostol, plasma concentration quickly reaches a peak level and then sinks rapidly, whereas after vaginal misoprostol, the peak concentration is reached slower, and plasma concentration also declines slowly [24]. A pharmacokinetic study by Tang et al., comparing plasma concentration after oral, vaginal, and sublingual application of misoprostol before first-trimester surgical abortion showed that highest peak-plasma concentrations are reached after sublingual application, and the peak concentration is also reached fastest after sublingual application [5]. Therefore, it can be hypothesized that the incidence of ADR correlates with the rapidity by which concentration of misoprostol increases in the blood and with the finally reached peak plasma concentration.

In our study, gastrointestinal ADR occurred significantly more frequently in women who received misoprostol orally compared to vaginally for cervical ripening (RR random = 1.9, CI 95%: 1.17-3.09). These results were confirmed by a Cochrane review conducted by Alfirevic et al., comparing oral vs. vaginal misoprostol for labour induction: nausea (RR = 1.06, CI 95%: 0.76-1.48), vomiting (RR = 1.16, CI 95%: 0.78-1.72), and diarrhoea (RR = 1.63, CI 95%: 0.87-3.06) [25].

Gastrointestinal ADR were also more frequent in women receiving oral misoprostol for the induction of abortion when compared to vaginal application (RR random = 1.42, CI 95%: 0.97-2.08), but this is not statistically significant. A Cochrane review conducted by Dodd et al. comparing vaginal vs. oral misoprostol for the induction of abortion in the second or third trimester confirmed that oral application causes more gastrointestinal ADR (nausea: RR = 0.69, CI 95%: 0.42-1.13; vomiting: RR = 0.71, CI 95%: 0.48-1.07; diarrhoea: RR = 0.88, CI 95%: 0.24-3.26) [23]. Another Cochrane review comparing vaginal vs. oral misoprostol for abortion induction under 24 weeks of gestation, conducted by Neilson et al., also resulted in less gastrointestinal ADR with vaginal misoprostol (nausea: RR = 0.63, CI 95%: 0.26-1.54; vomiting: RR = 0.36, CI 95%: 0.07-1.75; diarrhoea: RR = 0.21, CI 95%: 0.12-0.36) [26].

In our study we could show a statistically significant higher incidence of gastrointestinal ADR for sublingual vs. vaginal misoprostol for the indication abortion (RR random = 1.24, CI 95%: 1.02-1.51), however the difference was not significant for cervical ripening and labour induction (RR random = 1.67, CI 95%: 0.95-2.96). Dodd et al. compared sublingual vs. vaginal misoprostol for second or third-trimester abortions and described less vomiting (RR = 0.69, CI 95%: 0.35-1.33), but more diarrhoea (RR = 2.50, CI 95%: 0.51-12.30) after sublingual misoprostol [23].

Comparing the oral and sublingual mode of application we could show that gastrointestinal ADR were less frequent with oral misoprostol for cervical ripening and labour induction (RR random = 0.49, CI 95%: 0.08-3.06), but more frequent after abortion induction (RR random = 1.45, CI 95%: 0.73-2.87). However, both results are not significant. Dodd et al. found less vomiting (RR = 0.85, CI 95%: 0.42-1.71) and less diarrhoea (RR = 0.83, CI 95%: 0.27-2.56) after sublingual misoprostol compared to oral misoprostol for second or third trimester abortion [23].

In our study, fever and shivering occurred more frequently after oral as well as after sublingual application when compared to vaginal application in the indication cervical ripening (RR random = 1.06, CI 95%: 0.32-3.64 and 2,0 CI 95%: 0.82-4.90, respectively). The same applies to the indication abortion induction when sublingual vs. vaginal misoprostol are compared (RR random = 1.22, CI 95%: 0.91-1.62), but was not confirmed for oral vs. vaginal misoprostol (RR random = 0.98, CI 95%: 0.57-1.70). All these results are not statistically significant, however.

Serious Maternal ADR

Of the 126'477 women included in the study, receiving misoprostol for cervical ripening and labour induction or abortion induction, 67 experienced a dehiscence or rupture of the uterus. 26 of the 34 cases receiving misoprostol for cervical ripening and labour induction occurred after vaginal application of misoprostol, and only three cases after oral application. It would be interesting to find out whether this was merely due to the fact that the vaginal mode of application is more commonly used for this indication, or whether vaginal misoprostol really bears a higher risk of causing uterine rupture. There are only few meta-analyses comparing oral to vaginal misoprostol regarding the risk of uterine rupture in the current literature. In the Cochrane review conducted by Alfirevic et al. there was no case of uterine rupture in either group, so the risk could not be evaluated [25]. They postulated: "Some observational studies have reported a high uterine-rupture rate when vaginal misoprostol was given to women who have had previous cesarean sections. There is less evidence for oral misoprostol, but there were rupture rates of 10% (1 of 10) and 9.7% (4 of 41) in two studies that used oral misoprostol for labour induction with previous section." [25].

Maternal death occurred in 29 of the total of 126'477 women, of whom four received misoprostol for cervical ripening and labour induction, three for abortion induction, and 21 for the prevention or treatment of PPH. The reason for the much higher number of cases of women receiving misoprostol for the prevention or treatment of PPH is not clear, but it is presumably mainly influenced by the type and setting of the studies.

5.2 Delivery

When 25 vs. 50 µg vaginal misoprostol administered for cervical ripening and labour induction were compared, hyperstimulation syndrome occurred less frequently with the lower dose regimen (RR random = 0.61, CI 95%: 0.31-1.21). A Cochrane review conducted by Hofmeyr et al., comparing low vs. high dosages of vaginal misoprostol confirmed these results (16 trials, RR = 0.51, CI 95%: 0.37 to 0.69). When oral vs. vaginal misoprostol for cervical ripening and labour induction were compared, hyperstimulation syndrome occurred more frequently after oral (18.9% CI 95%: 17.7-20.0) than after vaginal (6.3% CI 95%: 5.9-6.7) application. Contradictory to these results, Hofmeyr et al. suggest a lower incidence of hyperstimulation syndrome with oral than with vaginal misoprostol (9% vs. 24.6%; RR = 0.37, CI 95%: 0.23-0.59) [27]. These results show that the incidence of hyperstimulation syndrome as the ADR seems to depend on the dose and the mode of application of misoprostol.

In our study we also tried to find out whether misoprostol is superior to other medicaments concerning the safety and efficacy in its use in obstetrics. The comparison of oral misoprostol vs. vaginal or cervical PGE2 (RR random = 0.96, CI 95%: 0.62-1.49) and vaginal misoprostol vs. oxytocin (RR random = 1.06, 0.49-2.28) resulted in no significant difference in the incidence of hyperstimulation syndrome. However, the incidence was slightly higher for vaginal misoprostol when compared to vaginal or cervical PGE2 (RR random = 1.31, CI 95%: 0.94-1.83). Hofmeyr et al. also show a higher incidence of hyperstimulation syndrome after vaginal misoprostol when compared to vaginal (31 trials, RR = 1.43, 95% CI 0.97 - 2.09) or cervical prostaglandins (20 trials, RR = 2.32, 95% CI 1.64 - 3.28) [27].

We could show a significantly lower risk for caesarean section with oral misoprostol vs. placebo (RR random = 0.61, CI 95%: 0.42-0.89), however this was not confirmed for vaginal misoprostol vs. placebo (RR random = 1.09, CI 95%: 0.68-1.74).

The use of oral misoprostol resulted in a significant lower caesarean section rate when compared to vaginal or cervical PGE 2 (RR = 0.84, CI 95%: 0.74-0.96). Hofmeyer et al. found a trend of reduction in caesarean section risk with vaginal misoprostol when compared to other vaginal prostaglandins (RR 0.95, 95%CI 0.87-1.03) and also when compared to oxytocin (RR 0.76, CI 95%: 0.60-0.96) [27].

5.3 Neonatal Outcome

Overall, signs of foetal distress were the most commonly observed ADR of the newborns.

The most evident difference in the incidence of signs of foetal distress was found when dosages of ≤300 µg vs. >300 µg of oral misoprostol (14.4 %, CI 95%: 13.0-15.9% vs. 19.0%,CI 95%: 17.6-20.5, respectively) were compared, which also confirms a certain dose-dependence.

Neonatal death occurred in four cases after oral and in 60 cases after vaginal application, but this is assumed to be related mainly to the fact that a much higher number of women with cervical ripening and labour induction received vaginal than oral misoprostol (48 vs. 21% of all 10'744 women in this indication).

The evaluation of the other neonatal ADR showed no significant difference in occurrences that could be related to the use of different dose regimens or application modes of misoprostol.

5.4 Strengths and Weaknesses of this Study

The selection of the studies was based mainly on the usage of misoprostol in its three main indications in pregnant women. Data from pro and retrospective studies, ranging from single-case reports to big multicenter RCTs, was included in the analysis. The primary aim was to avoid missing important information on rarely occurring ADR, namely uterine rupture and maternal death, after medication with misoprostol. This method resulted in an extensive amount of available data for evaluation, but also inevitably led to a remarkable heterogeneity in terms of quality of the collected data.

The analysis of the data concerning mothers and children was conducted solely by dividing it into three subgroups according to the three main indications. Further aspects of the mother (age weight, gravida, para, intact or ruptured membranes, previous caesarean section, comorbidities, etc.) or the foetus (sex, weight and size at birth, age at time of abortion, etc.) were not considered. Aspects such as the exact reason for treatment with misoprostol (e.g. cervical ripening prior to labour induction vs. prior to surgical termination or first vs. second-trimester abortion), exact gestational age, its status after caesarean section, or comorbidities of the mother were listed in the database, but were not evaluated in detail due to the great discrepancy of data, which would have made comparative analysis difficult. Furthermore, due to lack of information in some study reports, aspects such as source, dose, or mode of application of misoprostol could not be collected for all studies.

For these reasons, the study group was quite heterogeneous and could therefore only be characterised at a basic level.

Sometimes it was necessary to compare big study groups with small ones (for example, when oral and vaginal application were compared in the indications cervical ripening and labour induction and abortion induction), due to the fact that vaginal misoprostol was used more frequently in these indications; or when misoprostol alone was compared to the combination with oxytocin, because the number of women treated with misoprostol alone was much higher than the number treated with the combined regimen.

ADR were only evaluated if they were mentioned in the study report. If no ADR were mentioned at all, this was not interpreted as "no ADR", which could have made the apparent frequency of ADR too high.

ADR were condensed in different subgroups, e.g. nausea, vomiting, and diarrhoea were summarised under the term "gastrointestinal ADR". If a woman suffered from two gastrointestinal ADR at the same time, e.g. of nausea and vomiting or fever and shivering, this was therefore counted as two events of ADR, which also makes the apparent frequency too high.

Some ADR, such as fever or PPH, are very heterogeneously defined in the different studies. The exact definition is mentioned in the database, but was not considered in the analysis.

Abdominal cramping and pain is a very common ADR after medication with misoprostol, especially after the induction of first and second-trimester abortions. It would have been very interesting to evaluate this ADR, but great variations between the strength of pain based on the subjective sensation in each patient and the very heterogeneous methods of describing pain (e.g. according to different pain scores or by the height of dose of analgesics required) made it impossible to generate data in an evaluable, comparable form.

13 of the 59 described cases of uterine rupture and three of the 28 cases of maternal death after medication with misoprostol were described in case reports. That these cases were also included in the primary analysis of data may lead to the impression that these serious incidences were more common than they really are.

Of the 28 cases of maternal death, 21 occurred after medication for the indication prevention or treatment of PPH. Six of the cases were after treatment of PPH with misoprostol, which may be because the women were already in too critical condition after heavy blood loss to be saved by uterotonics. Another important fact is that a large number of studies concerning the use of misoprostol for the indication prevention or treatment of PPH were conducted in developing countries, often not even in a hospital, but at the women's home the medical setting was therefore very different from that in the other clinical studies.

5.5 Appraisal of the off-label Use by the Legal Authority (Swissmedic)

On 21st October, 2011, we had a meeting with three experts of Swissmedic in Berne (Mrs. Grimm, pharmacist; Mr. Stötter, physician and Mr. Kopp, jurist).

The primary aim of this work was to get misoprostol out of its off-label use, which we tried to achieve by showing its efficacy and safety as proven by a large amount of research data collected during the past 20 years. We showed that misoprostol is very frequently used in Switzerland and that its use is documented broadly and was tested in numerous clinical studies. Unfortunately, all this documentation was after all not extensive enough to be used for a request for the expansion for permission of misoprostol in its obstetrical indications. Our talk with Swissmedic showed that there are several problems, which make it impossible for us to apply for an expansion of permission solely based on the results from this work.

In the following, the main results of our long discussion shall be presented:

At the University Hospital of Zurich, misoprostol is used daily as a first-line drug in obstetrics. Therefore, the interest in an expansion of permission for Cytotec ® has increased in the past years. It would facilitate the use of the drug in Swiss hospitals, if the medical staff had the support and confirmation of the authorities, that the efficacy and safety of misoprostol is sufficiently documented.

However, the situation is quite different in other European countries like Germany and Italy, and also in Canada, where Cytotec ® has already been withdrawn from sale even for its labelled indication of the prevention and treatment of gastroduodenal ulcers. According to Mr. Stötter, it is only a matter of time until it is also withdrawn in other countries, such as the USA, Spain, the Netherlands, or Denmark.

Getting an expansion for misoprostol in its obstetrical indications is at this time impossible for several reasons: First, it would be necessary to limit oneself to one single indication and to indicate whether the original compound (Cytotec ®) or a self-produced form was used, which galenic form was used, which mode of application and which dose was used, etc. All this data would have to be gathered prospectively, meaning that we would be required to conduct studies by ourselves.

Secondly, Swissmedic itself is not able to expand the permission of a drug without a corresponding request by the drug's current patent holder. The holder of the drug must fulfil certain criteria, for instance he must have the authorisation to sell the drug. If the compound is already available on the open market (as is the case with Cytotec ®), only the holder may request a change of conditions of permission from Swissmedic. In such a case, it is the duty of the firm to produce and collect data to prove the efficacy and safety of its drug and to submit this data to Swissmedic.

It will therefore be absolutely necessary to find out whether the current patent holder of Cytotec ®, the American company Pfizer, is interested in getting an expansion of permission of misoprostol. If the company is interested, it could give us further advice concerning the information needed for Swissmedic and eventually even give us internal research data to prove the efficacy and safety of its drug.

The three experts agreed that this would be very difficult to manage, and they doubt that there is any interest from Pfizer to get an expansion of permission for Cytotec ®. On the one hand, Pfizer may be unwilling to take on the responsibility for a drug that is still suspected to carry a risk of causing serious adverse drug reactions in pregnant women, such as uterine rupture and maternal death (as recently occurred 2004 in Basle, where a woman died from the consequences of a uterine rupture after the induction of labour with misoprostol). On the other hand, misoprostol itself is a very cheap drug, so there is no financial incentive for Pfizer at all even less so, now that it might be or has already been withdrawn from sale in many other countries.

5.6 Conclusion and Outlook

This work shows that the number of sources of information generated over the last twenty years and more regarding the use of misoprostol in pregnancy, is extremely large. The analysis of all recorded data resulted in such an extensive number of results, that we were obliged to select only the most important ones to be presented in this work. Hopefully, no important results have escaped our notice. Nevertheless, it would be interesting to further analyse the remaining data.

The visit at the Swissmedic Institute in Berne and the lively debate on the use of misoprostol in obstetrics proved that, in spite of the widely conducted research on this topic, the discussion about its pros and cons is still going on.

The analysis of a selected number of studies concerning the use of misoprostol in its three main obstetrical indications cannot definitely solve the problem by giving a final statement about its efficacy and safety. On contrary, it proves the heterogeneity between pros and cons seen in the analysed studies. The comparison with other meta-analyses showed that most of the findings of our study correspond with the current state of research.

The description of cases with serious ADR showed that despite profound research on its efficacy and safety, the treatment with misoprostol is still fraught with a certain risk. This fact has gained even more relevance in light of a case of maternal death due to uterine rupture after labour induction with misoprostol at the University Hospital of Basle in 2004. The case reminds us, that women treated with misoprostol require well-managed and intensive monitoring, so that dangerous cases can be recognized, and intervention can be made at the right time. To draw a definitive conclusion, it would be necessary to compare the frequency of uterine dehiscence and rupture and of maternal death with other medications or without treatment.

Hopefully, this work is nevertheless successful in laying the ground for further and more detailed investigations, based on the considerable amount of available data. It would be very interesting to conduct further analyses of the data as proposed by Mr. Stötter and Mrs. Grimm from Swissmedic. The next step would hence be to establish contact with Pfizer, to ask whether there is any interest to expand the permission of Cytotec ® for obstetrical use, and then to find out which additional data is necessary to get this permission - the final aim being Swissmedic's approval for misoprostol for the licensed use in obstetrics in Switzerland.

6. References

6.1 Analysed Studies

Abbasi, N., N. Danish, et al. (2008). "Effectiveness and safety of vaginal misoprostol for induction of labour in unfavourable cervix in 3rd trimester." J Ayub Med Coll Abbottabad **20**(3): 33-35.

Abd-El-Maeboud, K. H., A. A. Ghazy, et al. (2008). "Effect of vaginal pH on the efficacy of vaginal misoprostol for induction of midtrimester abortion." J Obstet Gynaecol Res **34**(1): 78-84.

Abdel-Aleem, H., I. El-Nashar, et al. (2001). "Management of severe postpartum hemorrhage with misoprostol." Int J Gynaecol Obstet **72**(1): 75-76.

Abdellah, M. S., M. Hussien, et al. (2010). "Intravaginal administration of isosorbide mononitrate and misoprostol for cervical ripening and induction of labour: a randomized controlled trial." Arch Gynecol Obstet.

Abdul, M. A., U. N. Ibrahim, et al. (2007). "Efficacy and safety of misoprostol in induction of labour in a Nigerian tertiary hospital." West Afr J Med **26**(3): 213-216.

Abramovici, D., S. Goldwasser, et al. (1999). "A randomized comparison of oral misoprostol versus Foley catheter and oxytocin for induction of labor at term." Am J Obstet Gynecol **181**(5 Pt 1): 1108-1112.

Acharya, G., M. T. Al-Sammarai, et al. (2001). "A randomized, controlled trial comparing effect of oral misoprostol and intravenous syntocinon on intra-operative blood loss during cesarean section." Acta Obstet Gynecol Scand **80**(3): 245-250.

Adair, C. D., J. W. Weeks, et al. (1998). "Oral or vaginal misoprostol administration for induction of labor: a randomized, double-blind trial." Obstet Gynecol **92**(5): 810-813.

Adam, I., O. A. Hassan, et al. (2005). "Oral misoprostol vs. vaginal misoprostol for cervical ripening and labor induction." Int J Gynaecol Obstet **89**(2): 142-143.

Adekanmi, O. A., S. Purmessur, et al. (2001). "Intrauterine misoprostol for the treatment of severe recurrent atonic secondary postpartum haemorrhage." BJOG **108**(5): 541-542.

Adeniji, A. O., O. Olayemi, et al. (2006). "Intravaginal misoprostol versus transcervical Foley catheter in pre-induction cervical ripening." Int J Gynaecol Obstet **92**(2): 130-132.

Adeniji, A. O., O. Olayemi, et al. (2005). "Comparison of changes in pre-induction cervical factors' scores following ripening with transcervical foley catheter and intravaginal misoprostol." Afr J Med Med Sci **34**(4): 377-382.

Adeniji, A. O., O. Olayemi, et al. (2005). "Cervico-vaginal foetal fibronectin: a predictor of cervical response at pre-induction cervical ripening." West Afr J Med **24**(4): 334-337.

Adeniji, O. A., A. Oladokun, et al. (2005). "Pre-induction cervical ripening: transcervical foley catheter versus intravaginal misoprostol." J Obstet Gynaecol **25**(2): 134-139.

Afolabi, B. B., O. L. Oyeneyin, et al. (2005). "Intravaginal misoprostol versus Foley catheter for cervical ripening and induction of labor." Int J Gynaecol Obstet **89**(3): 263-267.

Afolabi, E. O., O. Kuti, et al. (2010). "Oral misoprostol versus intramuscular oxytocin in the active management of the third stage of labour." Singapore Med J **51**(3): 207-211.

Agarwal, N., A. Gupta, et al. (2003). "Six hourly vaginal misoprostol versus intracervical dinoprostone for cervical ripening and labor induction." J Obstet Gynaecol Res **29**(3): 147-151.

Akoury, H. A., M. E. Hannah, et al. (2004). "Randomized controlled trial of misoprostol for second-trimester pregnancy termination associated with fetal malformation." Am J Obstet Gynecol **190**(3): 755-762.

Al-Hussaini, T. K. (2001). "Uterine rupture in second trimester abortion in a grand multiparous woman. A complication of misoprostol and oxytocin." Eur J Obstet Gynecol Reprod Biol **96**(2): 218-219.

Al-Hussaini, T. K., S. A. Abdel-Aal, et al. (2003). "Oral misoprostol vs. intravenous oxytocin for labor induction in women with prelabor rupture of membranes at term." Int J Gynaecol Obstet **82**(1): 73-75.

Al-Taani, M. I. (2005). "Termination of second trimester, complicated gestation." East Mediterr Health J **11**(4): 657-662.

Al Inizi, S. A. and M. Ezimokhai (2003). "Vaginal misoprostol versus dinoprostone for the management of missed abortion." Int J Gynaecol Obstet **83**(1): 73-74.

Alsibiani, S. A. (2009). "Misoprostol for pregnancy termination in grand multiparous women with three cesarean deliveries." Int J Gynaecol Obstet **106**(3): 255-256.

Amant, F., B. Spitz, et al. (1999). "Misoprostol compared with methylergometrine for the prevention of postpartum haemorrhage: a double-blind randomised trial." Br J Obstet Gynaecol **106**(10): 1066-1070.

Aronsson, A., M. Bygdeman, et al. (2004). "Effects of misoprostol on uterine contractility following different routes of administration." Hum Reprod **19**(1): 81-84.

Aronsson, A., L. Helstrom, et al. (2004). "Sublingual compared with oral misoprostol for cervical dilatation prior to vacuum aspiration: a randomized comparison." Contraception **69**(2): 165-169.

Aronsson, A., A. K. Ulfgren, et al. (2005). "The effect of orally and vaginally administered misoprostol on inflammatory mediators and cervical ripening during early pregnancy." Contraception **72**(1): 33-39.

Arteaga-Troncoso, G., A. Villegas-Alvarado, et al. (2005). "Intracervical application of the nitric oxide donor isosorbide dinitrate for induction of cervical ripening: a randomised controlled trial to determine clinical efficacy and safety prior to first trimester surgical evacuation of retained products of conception." BJOG **112**(12): 1615-1619.

Ashok, P. W., H. Hamoda, et al. (2003). "Randomised controlled study comparing oral and vaginal misoprostol for cervical priming prior to surgical termination of pregnancy." BJOG **110**(12): 1057-1061.

Austin, S. C., L. Sanchez-Ramos, et al. (2010). "Labor induction with intravaginal misoprostol compared with the dinoprostone vaginal insert: a systematic review and metaanalysis." Am J Obstet Gynecol **202**(6): 624 e621-629.

Autry, A. M., E. C. Hayes, et al. (2002). "A comparison of medical induction and dilation and evacuation for second-trimester abortion." Am J Obstet Gynecol **187**(2): 393-397.

Ayad, I. A. (2002). "Vaginal misoprostol in managing premature rupture of membranes." East Mediterr Health J **8**(4-5): 515-520.

Ayati, S., F. V. Roudsari, et al. (2008). "Medical abortion at first trimester of pregnancy with misoprostol." Saudi Med J **29**(12): 1739-1742.

Ayaz, A., S. Saeed, et al. (2008). "Pre-labor rupture of membranes at term in patients with an unfavorable cervix: active versus conservative management." Taiwan J Obstet Gynecol **47**(2): 192-196.

Ayres-de-Campos, D., J. Teixeira-da-Silva, et al. (2000). "Vaginal misoprostol in the management of first-trimester missed abortions." Int J Gynaecol Obstet **71**(1): 53-57.

Ayudhaya, O. P., Y. Herabutya, et al. (2006). "A comparison of the efficacy of sublingual and oral misoprostol 400 microgram in the management of early pregnancy failure: a randomized controlled trial." J Med Assoc Thai **89 Suppl 4**: S5-10.

Bagratee, J. S., V. Khullar, et al. (2004). "A randomized controlled trial comparing medical and expectant management of first trimester miscarriage." Hum Reprod **19**(2): 266-271.

Balci, O., A. S. Mahmoud, et al. "Comparison of induction of labor with vaginal misoprostol plus oxytocin versus oxytocin alone in term primigravidae." J Matern Fetal Neonatal Med.

Balci, O., A. S. Mahmoud, et al. "Induction of labor with vaginal misoprostol plus oxytocin versus oxytocin alone." Int J Gynaecol Obstet **110**(1): 64-67.

Bamigboye, A. A., G. J. Hofmeyr, et al. (1998). "Rectal misoprostol in the prevention of postpartum hemorrhage: a placebo-controlled trial." Am J Obstet Gynecol **179**(4): 1043-1046.

Bamigboye, A. A., D. A. Merrell, et al. (1998). "Randomized comparison of rectal misoprostol with Syntometrine for management of third stage of labor." Acta Obstet Gynecol Scand **77**(2): 178-181.

Banos, A., M. Wolf, et al. (2007). "Frequency domain near-infrared spectroscopy of the uterine cervix during cervical ripening." Lasers Surg Med **39**(8): 641-646.

Barnhart, K. T., T. Bader, et al. (2004). "Hormone pattern after misoprostol administration for a nonviable first-trimester gestation." Fertil Steril **81**(4): 1099-1105.

Barrilleaux, P. S., J. A. Bofill, et al. (2002). "Cervical ripening and induction of labor with misoprostol, dinoprostone gel, and a Foley catheter: a randomized trial of 3 techniques." Am J Obstet Gynecol **186**(6): 1124-1129.

Bartha, J. L., R. Comino-Delgado, et al. (2000). "Oral misoprostol and intracervical dinoprostone for cervical ripening and labor induction: a randomized comparison." Obstet Gynecol **96**(3): 465-469.

Baruah, M. and G. M. Cohn (2008). "Efficacy of rectal misoprostol as second-line therapy for the treatment of primary postpartum hemorrhage." J Reprod Med **53**(3): 203-206.

Baskett, T. F., V. L. Persad, et al. (2007). "Misoprostol versus oxytocin for the reduction of postpartum blood loss." Int J Gynaecol Obstet **97**(1): 2-5.

Basu, J. K. and D. Basu (2009). "The management of failed second-trimester termination of pregnancy." Contraception **80**(2): 170-173.

Batioglu, S., E. Tonguc, et al. (1997). "Midtrimester termination of complicated pregnancy with oral misoprostol." Adv Contracept **13**(1): 55-61.

Bebbington, M. W., N. Kent, et al. (2002). "A randomized controlled trial comparing two protocols for the use of misoprostol in midtrimester pregnancy termination." Am J Obstet Gynecol **187**(4): 853-857.

Behrashi, M. and M. Mahdian (2008). "Vaginal versus oral misoprostol for second-trimester pregnancy termination: a randomized trial." Pak J Biol Sci **11**(21): 2505-2508.

Beigi, A., M. Kabiri, et al. (2003). "Cervical ripening with oral misoprostol at term." Int J Gynaecol Obstet **83**(3): 251-255.

Benchimol, M., J. Gondry, et al. (2001). "[Role of misoprostol in the delivery outcome]." J Gynecol Obstet Biol Reprod (Paris) **30**(6): 576-583.

Bennett, K. A., K. Butt, et al. (1998). "A masked randomized comparison of oral and vaginal administration of misoprostol for labor induction." Obstet Gynecol **92**(4 Pt 1): 481-486.

Bentov, Y., E. Sheiner, et al. (2004). "Misoprostol overdose during the first trimester of pregnancy." Eur J Obstet Gynecol Reprod Biol **115**(1): 108-109.

Berghahn, L., D. Christensen, et al. (2001). "Uterine rupture during second-trimester abortion associated with misoprostol." Obstet Gynecol **98**(5 Pt 2): 976-977.

Berkley, E., C. Meng, et al. (2007). "Success rates with low dose misoprostol before induction of labor for nulliparas with severe preeclampsia at various gestational ages." J Matern Fetal Neonatal Med **20**(11): 825-831.

Bernardi, P., C. Graziadio, et al. (2010). "Fibular dimelia and mirror polydactyly of the foot in a girl presenting additional features of the VACTERL association." Sao Paulo Med J **128**(2): 99-101.

Beucher, G. (2010). "[Management of spontaneous miscarriage in the first trimester]." J Gynecol Obstet Biol Reprod (Paris) **39**(3 Suppl): F3-10.

Beucher, G., S. Baume, et al. (2004). "[Medical treatment of early spontaneous miscarriages: a prospective study of outpatient management using misoprostol]." J Gynecol Obstet Biol Reprod (Paris) **33**(5): 401-406.

Bhattacharjee, N., R. P. Ganguly, et al. (2007). "Misoprostol for termination of mid-trimester post-Caesarean pregnancy." Aust N Z J Obstet Gynaecol **47**(1): 23-25.

Bhattacharjee, N., S. P. Saha, et al. (2008). "A randomised comparative study on sublingual versus vaginal administration of misoprostol for termination of pregnancy between 13 to 20 weeks." Aust N Z J Obstet Gynaecol **48**(2): 165-171.

Bhattacharyya, S. K., J. Mukherji, et al. (2006). "Two regimens of vaginal misoprostol in second trimester termination of pregnancy: a prospective randomised trial." Acta Obstet Gynecol Scand **85**(12): 1458-1462.

Bhullar, A., S. J. Carlan, et al. (2004). "Buccal misoprostol to decrease blood loss after vaginal delivery: a randomized trial." Obstet Gynecol **104**(6): 1282-1288.

Billings, D. L. (2004). "Misoprostol alone for early medical abortion in a Latin American clinic setting." Reprod Health Matters **12**(24 Suppl): 57-64.

Bique, C., A. Bugalho, et al. (1999). "Labor induction by vaginal misoprostol in grand multiparous women." Acta Obstet Gynecol Scand **78**(3): 198-201.

Bique, C., M. Usta, et al. (2007). "Comparison of misoprostol and manual vacuum aspiration for the treatment of incomplete abortion." Int J Gynaecol Obstet **98**(3): 222-226.

Blanchard, K., T. Shochet, et al. (2005). "Misoprostol alone for early abortion: an evaluation of seven potential regimens." Contraception **72**(2): 91-97.

Blanchard, K., S. Taneepanichskul, et al. (2004). "Two regimens of misoprostol for treatment of incomplete abortion." Obstet Gynecol **103**(5 Pt 1): 860-865.

Blanchette, H. A., S. Nayak, et al. (1999). "Comparison of the safety and efficacy of intravaginal misoprostol (prostaglandin E1) with those of dinoprostone (prostaglandin E2) for cervical ripening and induction of labor in a community hospital." Am J Obstet Gynecol **180**(6 Pt 1): 1551-1559.

Blohm, F., B. E. Friden, et al. (2005). "A randomised double blind trial comparing misoprostol or placebo in the management of early miscarriage." BJOG **112**(8): 1090-1095.

Blum, J., B. Winikoff, et al. (2010). "Treatment of post-partum haemorrhage with sublingual misoprostol versus oxytocin in women receiving prophylactic oxytocin: a double-blind, randomised, non-inferiority trial." Lancet **375**(9710): 217-223.

Bolnick, J. M., M. D. Velazquez, et al. (2004). "Randomized trial between two active labor management protocols in the presence of an unfavorable cervix." Am J Obstet Gynecol **190**(1): 124-128.

Bond, G. R. and A. Van Zee (1994). "Overdosage of misoprostol in pregnancy." Am J Obstet Gynecol **171**(2): 561-562.

Borgatta, L., A. Y. Chen, et al. (2005). "A randomized clinical trial of the addition of laminaria to misoprostol and hypertonic saline for second-trimester induction abortion." Contraception **72**(5): 358-361.

Borgatta, L., B. Mullally, et al. (2004). "Misoprostol as the primary agent for medical abortion in a low-income urban setting." Contraception **70**(2): 121-126.

Borgatta, L., R. Sayegh, et al. (2009). "Cervical obstruction complicating second-trimester abortion: treatment with misoprostol." Obstet Gynecol **113**(2 Pt 2): 548-550.

Boza, A. V., R. G. de Leon, et al. (2008). "Misoprostol preferable to ethacridine lactate for abortions at 13-20 weeks of pregnancy: Cuban experience." Reprod Health Matters **16**(31 Suppl): 189-195.

Bricker, L., H. Peden, et al. (2008). "Titrated low-dose vaginal and/or oral misoprostol to induce labour for prelabour membrane rupture: a randomised trial." BJOG **115**(12): 1503-1511.

Buccellato, C. A., C. S. Stika, et al. (2000). "A randomized trial of misoprostol versus extra-amniotic sodium chloride infusion with oxytocin for induction of labor." Am J Obstet Gynecol **182**(5): 1039-1044.

Bugalho, A., C. Bique, et al. (1993). "Pregnancy interruption by vaginal misoprostol." Gynecol Obstet Invest **36**(4): 226-229.

Bugalho, A., C. Bique, et al. (1994). "Application of vaginal misoprostol before cervical dilatation to facilitate first-trimester pregnancy interruption." Obstet Gynecol **83**(5 Pt 1): 729-731.

Bugalho, A., C. Bique, et al. (1993). "The effectiveness of intravaginal misoprostol (Cytotec) in inducing abortion after eleven weeks of pregnancy." Stud Fam Plann **24**(5): 319-323.

Bugalho, A., C. Bique, et al. (1994). "Induction of labor with intravaginal misoprostol in intrauterine fetal death." Am J Obstet Gynecol **171**(2): 538-541.

Bugalho, A., C. Bique, et al. (1996). "Uterine evacuation by vaginal misoprostol after second trimester pregnancy interruption." Acta Obstet Gynecol Scand **75**(3): 270-273.

Bugalho, A., A. Daniel, et al. (2001). "Misoprostol for prevention of postpartum hemorrhage." Int J Gynaecol Obstet **73**(1): 1-6.

Bugalho, A., A. Faundes, et al. (1996). "Evaluation of the effectiveness of vaginal misoprostol to induce first trimester abortion." Contraception **53**(4): 244-246.

Bugalho, A., S. Mocumbi, et al. (2000). "Termination of pregnancies of <6 weeks gestation with a single dose of 800 microg of vaginal misoprostol." Contraception **61**(1): 47-50.

Burnett, M. A., C. A. Corbett, et al. (2005). "A randomized trial of laminaria tents versus vaginal misoprostol for cervical ripening in first trimester surgical abortion." J Obstet Gynaecol Can **27**(1): 38-42.

Buser, D., G. Mora, et al. (1997). "A randomized comparison between misoprostol and dinoprostone for cervical ripening and labor induction in patients with unfavorable cervices." Obstet Gynecol **89**(4): 581-585.

Butt, K. D., K. A. Bennett, et al. (1999). "Randomized comparison of oral misoprostol and oxytocin for labor induction in term prelabor membrane rupture." Obstet Gynecol **94**(6): 994-999.

Cakir, L., B. Dilbaz, et al. (2005). "Comparison of oral and vaginal misoprostol for cervical ripening before manual vacuum aspiration of first trimester pregnancy under local anesthesia: a randomized placebo-controlled study." Contraception **71**(5): 337-342.

Calder, A. A., A. D. Loughney, et al. (2008). "Induction of labour in nulliparous and multiparous women: a UK, multicentre, open-label study of intravaginal misoprostol in comparison with dinoprostone." BJOG **115**(10): 1279-1288.

Caliskan, E., B. Dilbaz, et al. (2003). "Oral misoprostol for the third stage of labor: a randomized controlled trial." Obstet Gynecol **101**(5 Pt 1): 921-928.

Caliskan, E., S. Dilbaz, et al. (2005). "Randomized comparison of 3 misoprostol protocols for abortion induction at 13-20 weeks of gestation." J Reprod Med **50**(3): 173-180.

Caliskan, E., S. Dilbaz, et al. (2004). "Unsucessful labour induction in women with unfavourable cervical scores: predictors and management." <u>Aust N Z J Obstet Gynaecol</u> **44**(6): 562-567.

Caliskan, E., E. Doger, et al. (2009). "Sublingual misoprostol 100 microgram versus 200 microgram for second trimester abortion: a randomised trial." <u>Eur J Contracept Reprod Health Care</u> **14**(1): 55-60.

Caliskan, E., T. Filiz, et al. (2007). "Sublingual versus vaginal misoprostol for cervical ripening PRIOR TO manual vacuum aspiration under local anaesthesia: a randomized study." <u>Eur J Contracept Reprod Health Care</u> **12**(4): 372-377.

Caliskan, E., M. M. Meydanli, et al. (2002). "Is rectal misoprostol really effective in the treatment of third stage of labor? A randomized controlled trial." <u>Am J Obstet Gynecol</u> **187**(4): 1038-1045.

Carbonell Esteve, J. L., J. M. Mari, et al. (2006). "Sublingual versus vaginal misoprostol (400 microg) for cervical priming in first-trimester abortion: a randomized trial." <u>Contraception</u> **74**(4): 328-333.

Carbonell Esteve, J. L., L. Varela, et al. (1998). "Vaginal misoprostol for late first trimester abortion." <u>Contraception</u> **57**(5): 329-333.

Carbonell, J. L., J. Rodriguez, et al. (2001). "Vaginal misoprostol 1000 microg for early abortion." <u>Contraception</u> **63**(3): 131-136.

Carbonell, J. L., J. Rodriguez, et al. (2004). "Vaginal misoprostol 800 microg every 12 h for second-trimester abortion." <u>Contraception</u> **70**(1): 55-60.

Carbonell, J. L., J. Rodriguez, et al. (2003). "Oral and vaginal misoprostol 800 microg every 8 h for early abortion." <u>Contraception</u> **67**(6): 457-462.

Carbonell, J. L., M. A. Torres, et al. (2008). "Second-trimester pregnancy termination with 600-microg vs. 400-microg vaginal misoprostol and systematic curettage postexpulsion: a randomized trial." <u>Contraception</u> **77**(1): 50-55.

Carbonell, J. L., L. Valera, et al. (1998). "Vaginal misoprostol for early second-trimester abortion." <u>Eur J Contracept Reprod Health Care</u> **3**(2): 93-98.

Carbonell, J. L., L. Varela, et al. (1997). "The use of misoprostol for termination of early pregnancy." Contraception **55**(3): 165-168.

Carbonell, J. L., L. Varela, et al. (1997). "The use of misoprostol for abortion at < or = 9 weeks' gestation." Eur J Contracept Reprod Health Care **2**(3): 181-185.

Carbonell, J. L., L. Varela, et al. (2000). "Vaginal misoprostol 600 microg for early abortion." Eur J Contracept Reprod Health Care **5**(1): 46-51.

Carbonell, J. L., L. Varela, et al. (1999). "Vaginal misoprostol for abortion at 10-13 weeks' gestation." Eur J Contracept Reprod Health Care **4**(1): 35-40.

Carbonell, J. L., A. Velazco, et al. (2001). "Oral versus vaginal misoprostol for cervical priming in first-trimester abortion: a randomized trial." Eur J Contracept Reprod Health Care **6**(3): 134-140.

Carbonell, J. L., A. Velazco, et al. (2001). "Misoprostol for abortion at 9-12 weeks' gestation in adolescents." Eur J Contracept Reprod Health Care **6**(1): 39-45.

Carlan, S. J., D. Blust, et al. (2002). "Buccal versus intravaginal misoprostol administration for cervical ripening." Am J Obstet Gynecol **186**(2): 229-233.

Carlan, S. J., S. Bouldin, et al. (2001). "Safety and efficacy of misoprostol orally and vaginally: a randomized trial." Obstet Gynecol **98**(1): 107-112.

Carlan, S. J., S. Bouldin, et al. (1997). "Extemporaneous preparation of misoprostol gel for cervical ripening: a randomized trial." Obstet Gynecol **90**(6): 911-915.

Castaneda, C. S., J. C. Izquierdo Puente, et al. (2005). "Misoprostol dose selection in a controlled-release vaginal insert for induction of labor in nulliparous women." Am J Obstet Gynecol **193**(3 Pt 2): 1071-1075.

Cecatti, J. G., R. P. Tedesco, et al. (2006). "Effectiveness and safety of a new vaginal misoprostol product specifically labeled for cervical ripening and labor induction." Acta Obstet Gynecol Scand **85**(6): 706-711.

Celentano, C., F. Prefumo, et al. (2004). "Oral misoprostol vs. vaginal gemeprost prior to surgical termination of pregnancy in nulliparae." Acta Obstet Gynecol Scand **83**(8): 764-768.

Chambers, D. G. and E. C. Mulligan (2009). "Treatment of suction termination of pregnancy-retained products with misoprostol markedly reduces the repeat operation rate." Aust N Z J Obstet Gynaecol **49**(5): 551-553.

Chambers, D. G., E. C. Mulligan, et al. (2009). "Comparison of four perioperative misoprostol regimens for surgical termination of first-trimester pregnancy." Int J Gynaecol Obstet **107**(3): 211-215.

Chan, C. C., O. S. Tang, et al. (2005). "Intracervical sodium nitroprusside versus vaginal misoprostol in first trimester surgical termination of pregnancy: a randomized double-blinded controlled trial." Hum Reprod **20**(3): 829-833.

Chandhiok, N., B. S. Dhillon, et al. (2006). "Oral misoprostol for prevention of postpartum hemorrhage by paramedical workers in India." Int J Gynaecol Obstet **92**(2): 170-175.

Chang, C. H. and F. M. Chang (1997). "Randomized comparison of misoprostol and dinoprostone for preinduction cervical ripening and labor induction." J Formos Med Assoc **96**(5): 366-369.

Chang, D. W., M. D. Velazquez, et al. (2005). "Vaginal misoprostol for cervical ripening at term: comparison of outpatient vs. inpatient administration." J Reprod Med **50**(10): 735-739.

Chang, Y. K., W. H. Chen, et al. (2003). "Intracervical misoprostol and prostaglandin E2 for labor induction." Int J Gynaecol Obstet **80**(1): 23-28.

Chanrachakul, B., A. Chittachareon, et al. (2002). "Cephalocentesis with the modified Smellie's perforator." Int J Gynaecol Obstet **76**(2): 203-206.

Chanrachakul, B., Y. Herabutya, et al. (2002). "Randomized trial of isosorbide mononitrate versus misoprostol for cervical ripening at term." Int J Gynaecol Obstet **78**(2): 139-145.

Charoenkul, S. and M. Sripramote (2000). "A randomized comparison of one single dose of vaginal 50 microg misoprostol with 3 mg dinoprostone in pre-induction cervical ripening." J Med Assoc Thai **83**(9): 1026-1034.

Chaudhuri, P., G. B. Banerjee, et al. (2010). "Rectally administered misoprostol versus intravenous oxytocin infusion during cesarean delivery to reduce intraoperative and postoperative blood loss." Int J Gynaecol Obstet **109**(1): 25-29.

Chaudhuri, S., P. K. Banerjee, et al. (2010). "A comparison of two regimens of misoprostol for second trimester medical termination of pregnancy: a randomized trial." Trop Doct **40**(3): 144-148.

Chen, D. C., S. S. Yuan, et al. (2005). "Urinary cyclic guanosine 3',5'-monophosphate and cyclic adenosine 3',5'-monophosphate changes in spontaneous and induced onset active labor." Acta Obstet Gynecol Scand **84**(11): 1081-1086.

Chen, F. C., A. Bergann, et al. (2008). "Isosorbide mononitrate vaginal gel versus misoprostol vaginal gel versus Dilapan-S for cervical ripening before first trimester curettage." Eur J Obstet Gynecol Reprod Biol **138**(2): 176-179.

Chen, M., J. C. Shih, et al. (1999). "Separation of cesarean scar during second-trimester intravaginal misoprostol abortion." Obstet Gynecol **94**(5 Pt 2): 840.

Cheng, S. Y., C. S. Hsue, et al. (2010). "Comparison of labor induction with titrated oral misoprostol solution between nulliparous and multiparous women." J Obstet Gynaecol Res **36**(1): 72-78.

Cheng, S. Y., H. Ming, et al. (2008). "Titrated oral compared with vaginal misoprostol for labor induction: a randomized controlled trial." Obstet Gynecol **111**(1): 119-125.

Cheung, P. C., E. L. Yeo, et al. (2006). "Oral misoprostol for induction of labor in prelabor rupture of membranes (PROM) at term: a randomized control trial." Acta Obstet Gynecol Scand **85**(9): 1128-1133.

Cheung, W., O. S. Tang, et al. (2003). "Pilot study on the use of sublingual misoprostol in termination of pregnancy up to 7 weeks gestation." Contraception **68**(2): 97-99.

Chhabra, S. and C. Tickoo (2008). "Low-dose sublingual misoprostol versus methylergometrine for active management of the third stage of labor." J Obstet Gynaecol Res **34**(5): 820-823.

Chitaishvili, D. and T. Asatiani (2007). "Sublingual misoprostol prior to manual vacuum aspiration for reducing blood loss at 8-12 weeks of gestation: a randomized double-blind placebo-controlled study." Georgian Med News(152): 26-30.

Chong, Y. S., S. Chua, et al. (1997). "Severe hyperthermia following oral misoprostol in the immediate postpartum period." Obstet Gynecol **90**(4 Pt 2): 703-704.

Choo, W. L., S. Chua, et al. (1998). "Correlation of change in uterine activity to blood loss in the third stage of labour." Gynecol Obstet Invest **46**(3): 178-180.

Chung, J. H., W. H. Huang, et al. (2003). "A prospective randomized controlled trial that compared misoprostol, Foley catheter, and combination misoprostol-Foley catheter for labor induction." Am J Obstet Gynecol **189**(4): 1031-1035.

Chung, T., P. Leung, et al. (1997). "A medical approach to management of spontaneous abortion using misoprostol. Extending misoprostol treatment to a maximum of 48 hours can further improve evacuation of retained products of conception in spontaneous abortion." Acta Obstet Gynecol Scand **76**(3): 248-251.

Chung, T. K., D. T. Lee, et al. (1999). "Spontaneous abortion: a randomized, controlled trial comparing surgical evacuation with conservative management using misoprostol." Fertil Steril **71**(6): 1054-1059.

Coelho, H. L., A. C. Teixeira, et al. (1994). "Misoprostol: the experience of women in Fortaleza, Brazil." Contraception **49**(2): 101-110.

Coelho, H. L., A. C. Teixeira, et al. (1993). "Misoprostol and illegal abortion in Fortaleza, Brazil." Lancet **341**(8855): 1261-1263.

Coles, M. S. and L. P. Koenigs (2007). "Self-induced medical abortion in an adolescent." J Pediatr Adolesc Gynecol **20**(2): 93-95.

Collingham, J. P., K. C. Fuh, et al. (2010). "Oral misoprostol and vaginal isosorbide mononitrate for labor induction: a randomized controlled trial." Obstet Gynecol **116**(1): 121-126.

Colon, I., K. Clawson, et al. (2005). "Prospective randomized clinical trial of inpatient cervical ripening with stepwise oral misoprostol vs vaginal misoprostol." <u>Am J Obstet Gynecol</u> **192**(3): 747-752.

Cook, C. M., B. Spurrett, et al. (1999). "A randomized clinical trial comparing oral misoprostol with synthetic oxytocin or syntometrine in the third stage of labour." <u>Aust N Z J Obstet Gynaecol</u> **39**(4): 414-419.

Costa, S. H. and M. P. Vessey (1993). "Misoprostol and illegal abortion in Rio de Janeiro, Brazil." <u>Lancet</u> **341**(8855): 1258-1261.

Coughlin, L. B., D. Roberts, et al. (2004). "Medical management of first trimester incomplete miscarriage using misoprostol." <u>J Obstet Gynaecol</u> **24**(1): 67-68.

Crane, J. M., T. Delaney, et al. (2004). "Predictors of successful labor induction with oral or vaginal misoprostol." <u>J Matern Fetal Neonatal Med</u> **15**(5): 319-323.

Crane, J. M., T. Delaney, et al. (2003). "Oral misoprostol for premature rupture of membranes at term." <u>Am J Obstet Gynecol</u> **189**(3): 720-724.

Creinin, M. D., B. Harwood, et al. (2004). "Endometrial thickness after misoprostol use for early pregnancy failure." <u>Int J Gynaecol Obstet</u> **86**(1): 22-26.

Creinin, M. D., R. Moyer, et al. (1997). "Misoprostol for medical evacuation of early pregnancy failure." <u>Obstet Gynecol</u> **89**(5 Pt 1): 768-772.

Dabash, R., M. C. Ramadan, et al. (2010). "A randomized controlled trial of 400-mug sublingual misoprostol versus manual vacuum aspiration for the treatment of incomplete abortion in two Egyptian hospitals." <u>Int J Gynaecol Obstet</u> **111**(2): 131-135.

Daisley, H., Jr. (2000). "Maternal mortality following the use of misoprostol." <u>Med Sci Law</u> **40**(1): 78-82.

Dallenbach, P., M. Boulvain, et al. (2003). "Oral misoprostol or vaginal dinoprostone for labor induction: a randomized controlled trial." <u>Am J Obstet Gynecol</u> **188**(1): 162-167.

Danielsson, K. G., L. Marions, et al. (1999). "Comparison between oral and vaginal administration of misoprostol on uterine contractility." Obstet Gynecol **93**(2): 275-280.

Dao, B., J. Blum, et al. (2007). "Is misoprostol a safe, effective and acceptable alternative to manual vacuum aspiration for postabortion care? Results from a randomised trial in Burkina Faso, West Africa." BJOG **114**(11): 1368-1375.

Daponte, A., G. Nzewenga, et al. (2006). "The use of vaginal misoprostol for second-trimester pregnancy termination in women with previous single cesarean section." Contraception **74**(4): 324-327.

Daponte, A., G. Nzewenga, et al. (2007). "Pregnancy termination using vaginal misoprostol in women with more than one caesarean section." J Obstet Gynaecol **27**(6): 597-600.

Daskalakis, G., N. Papantoniou, et al. (2005). "Sonographic findings and surgical management of a uterine rupture associated with the use of misoprostol during second-trimester abortion." J Ultrasound Med **24**(11): 1565-1568.

Daskalakis, G. J., S. A. Mesogitis, et al. (2005). "Misoprostol for second trimester pregnancy termination in women with prior caesarean section." BJOG **112**(1): 97-99.

David, M. and F. C. Chen (2005). "Comparison of isosorbide mononitrate (Mono Mack) and misoprostol (Cytotec) for cervical ripening in the first trimester missed abortion." Arch Gynecol Obstet **273**(3): 144-145.

Davis, A. R., S. K. Hendlish, et al. (2007). "Bleeding patterns after misoprostol vs surgical treatment of early pregnancy failure: results from a randomized trial." Am J Obstet Gynecol **196**(1): 31 e31-37.

Davis, A. R., C. M. Robilotto, et al. (2004). "Bleeding patterns after vaginal misoprostol for treatment of early pregnancy failure." Hum Reprod **19**(7): 1655-1658.

De, A., R. Bagga, et al. (2006). "The routine use of oxytocin after oral misoprostol for labour induction in women with an unfavourable cervix is not of benefit." Aust N Z J Obstet Gynaecol **46**(4): 323-329.

de Aquino, M. M. and J. G. Cecatti (2003). "Misoprostol versus oxytocin for labor induction in term and post-term pregnancy: randomized controlled trial." Sao Paulo Med J **121**(3): 102-106.

de Jonge, E. T., R. Jewkes, et al. (2000). "Randomised controlled trial of the efficacy of misoprostol used as a cervical ripening agent prior to termination of pregnancy in the first trimester." S Afr Med J **90**(3): 256-262.

de Jonge, E. T., J. D. Makin, et al. (1995). "Randomised clinical trial of medical evacuation and surgical curettage for incomplete miscarriage." BMJ **311**(7006): 662.

Demetroulis, C., E. Saridogan, et al. (2001). "A prospective randomized control trial comparing medical and surgical treatment for early pregnancy failure." Hum Reprod **16**(2): 365-369.

Denguezli, W., A. Trimech, et al. (2007). "Efficacy and safety of six hourly vaginal misoprostol versus intracervical dinoprostone: a randomized controlled trial." Arch Gynecol Obstet **276**(2): 119-124.

Derman, R. J., B. S. Kodkany, et al. (2006). "Oral misoprostol in preventing postpartum haemorrhage in resource-poor communities: a randomised controlled trial." Lancet **368**(9543): 1248-1253.

Dickinson, J. E. (2004). "Late pregnancy termination within a legislated medical environment." Aust N Z J Obstet Gynaecol **44**(4): 337-341.

Dickinson, J. E. (2005). "Misoprostol for second-trimester pregnancy termination in women with a prior cesarean delivery." Obstet Gynecol **105**(2): 352-356.

Dickinson, J. E. and D. A. Doherty (2009). "Factors influencing the duration of pregnancy termination with vaginal misoprostol for fetal abnormality." Prenat Diagn **29**(5): 520-524.

Dickinson, J. E. and D. A. Doherty (2009). "Optimization of third-stage management after second-trimester medical pregnancy termination." Am J Obstet Gynecol **201**(3): 303 e301-307.

Dickinson, J. E. and S. F. Evans (2002). "The optimization of intravaginal misoprostol dosing schedules in second-trimester pregnancy termination." Am J Obstet Gynecol **186**(3): 470-474.

Dickinson, J. E. and S. F. Evans (2003). "A comparison of oral misoprostol with vaginal misoprostol administration in second-trimester pregnancy termination for fetal abnormality." Obstet Gynecol **101**(6): 1294-1299.

Dickinson, J. E., M. Godfrey, et al. (1998). "Efficacy of intravaginal misoprostol in second-trimester pregnancy termination: a randomized controlled trial." J Matern Fetal Med **7**(3): 115-119.

Dilbaz, S., E. Caliskan, et al. (2004). "Frequent low-dose misoprostol for termination of second-trimester pregnancy." Eur J Contracept Reprod Health Care **9**(1): 11-15.

Dilek, T. U., A. Doruk, et al. (2011). "Effect of cervical length on second trimester pregnancy termination." J Obstet Gynaecol Res.

Ding, D. C., H. Y. Su, et al. (2003). "Intravaginal and intracervical misoprostol for cervical ripening of labor in primiparas." Int J Gynaecol Obstet **82**(2): 209-211.

Diop, A., S. Raghavan, et al. (2009). "Two routes of administration for misoprostol in the treatment of incomplete abortion: a randomized clinical trial." Contraception **79**(6): 456-462.

Diro, M., A. Adra, et al. (1999). "A double-blind randomized trial of two dose regimens of misoprostol for cervical ripening and labor induction." J Matern Fetal Med **8**(3): 114-118.

Dodd, J., L. O'Brien, et al. (2005). "Misoprostol for second and third trimester termination of pregnancy: a review of practice at the Women's and Children's Hospital, Adelaide, Australia." Aust N Z J Obstet Gynaecol **45**(1): 25-29.

Dodd, J. M., C. A. Crowther, et al. (2006). "Morning compared with evening induction of labor: a nested randomized controlled trial. A nested randomized controlled trial." Obstet Gynecol **108**(2): 350-360.

Duhan, N., S. Gupta, et al. (2010). "Comparison of isosorbide mononitrate and misoprostol for cervical ripening in termination of pregnancy between 8 and 12 weeks: a randomized controlled trial." Arch Gynecol Obstet.

Durocher, J., J. Bynum, et al. (2010). "High fever following postpartum administration of sublingual misoprostol." BJOG **117**(7): 845-852.

Edelman, A. B., J. G. Buckmaster, et al. (2006). "Cervical preparation using laminaria with adjunctive buccal misoprostol before second-trimester dilation and evacuation procedures: a randomized clinical trial." Am J Obstet Gynecol **194**(2): 425-430.

Edwards, D., R. E. Aitken, et al. (1994). "Predilatation of the cervix before suction curettage for therapeutic abortion in early pregnancy." Aust N Z J Obstet Gynaecol **34**(1): 103-104.

Edwards, R. K. and S. M. Sims (2005). "Outcomes of second-trimester pregnancy terminations with misoprostol: comparing 2 regimens." Am J Obstet Gynecol **193**(2): 544-548; author reply 548-550.

Eftekhari, N., M. Doroodian, et al. (2009). "The effect of sublingual misoprostol versus intravenous oxytocin in reducing bleeding after caesarean section." J Obstet Gynaecol **29**(7): 633-636.

Ekele, B. A., D. C. Nnadi, et al. (2007). "Misoprostol use for cervical ripening and induction of labour in a Nigerian teaching hospital." Niger J Clin Pract **10**(3): 234-237.

Ekerhovd, E., N. Radulovic, et al. (2003). "Gemeprost versus misoprostol for cervical priming before first-trimester abortion: a randomized controlled trial." Obstet Gynecol **101**(4): 722-725.

El-Baradie, S. M., M. H. El-Said, et al. (2008). "Endometrial thickness and serum beta-hCG as predictors of the effectiveness of oral misoprostol in early pregnancy failure." J Obstet Gynaecol Can **30**(10): 877-881.

el-Refaey, H., L. Calder, et al. (1994). "Cervical priming with prostaglandin E1 analogues, misoprostol and gemeprost." Lancet **343**(8907): 1207-1209.

El-Refaey, H., R. Nooh, et al. (2000). "The misoprostol third stage of labour study: a randomised controlled comparison between orally administered misoprostol and standard management." BJOG **107**(9): 1104-1110.

el-Refaey, H., P. O'Brien, et al. (1997). "Use of oral misoprostol in the prevention of postpartum haemorrhage." Br J Obstet Gynaecol **104**(3): 336-339.

El-Sherbiny, M. T., I. H. El-Gharieb, et al. (2001). "Vaginal misoprostol for induction of labor: 25 vs. 50 microg dose regimen." Int J Gynaecol Obstet **72**(1): 25-30.

Elhassan, E. M., M. S. Abubaker, et al. (2008). "Sublingual compared with oral and vaginal misoprostol for termination of pregnancy with second-trimester fetal demise." Int J Gynaecol Obstet **100**(1): 82-83.

Elhassan, E. M., O. A. Mirghani, et al. (2005). "Cervical ripening and labor induction with 25 microg vs. 50 microg of intravaginal misoprostol." Int J Gynaecol Obstet **90**(3): 234-235.

Elhassan, M., O. A. Mirghani, et al. (2004). "Intravaginal misoprostol vs. dinoprostone as cervical ripening and labor-inducing agents." Int J Gynaecol Obstet **85**(3): 285-286.

Ellis, S. C., N. Kapp, et al. (2010). "Randomized trial of buccal versus vaginal misoprostol for induction of second trimester abortion." Contraception **81**(5): 441-445.

ElSedeek, M., E. E. Awad, et al. (2009). "Evaluation of postpartum blood loss after misoprostol-induced labour." BJOG **116**(3): 431-435.

Elsheikh, A., A. Antsaklis, et al. (2001). "Use of misoprostol for the termination of second trimester pregnancies." Arch Gynecol Obstet **265**(4): 204-206.

Enakpene, C. A., I. O. Morhason-Bello, et al. (2007). "Oral misoprostol for the prevention of primary post-partum hemorrhage during third stage of labor." J Obstet Gynaecol Res **33**(6): 810-817.

Eng, N. S. and A. C. Guan (1997). "Comparative study of intravaginal misoprostol with gemeprost as an abortifacient in second trimester missed abortion." Aust N Z J Obstet Gynaecol **37**(3): 331-334.

Escudero, F. and H. Contreras (1997). "A comparative trial of labor induction with misoprostol versus oxytocin." Int J Gynaecol Obstet **57**(2): 139-143.

Escumalha, M., C. Gouveia, et al. (2005). "Neonatal morbidity and outcome of live born premature babies after attempted illegal abortion with misoprostol." Pediatr Nurs **31**(3): 228-231.

Esteve, J. L., L. Varela, et al. (1999). "Early abortion with 800 micrograms of misoprostol by the vaginal route." Contraception **59**(4): 219-225.

Ezechi, O. C., B. K. Kalu, et al. (2004). "Vaginal misoprostol induction of labour: a Nigerian hospital experience." J Obstet Gynaecol **24**(3): 239-242.

Fadalla, F. A., O. A. Mirghani, et al. (2004). "Oral misoprostol vs. vaginal misoprostol for termination of pregnancy with intrauterine fetal demise in the second-trimester." Int J Gynaecol Obstet **86**(1): 52-53.

Farah, L. A., L. Sanchez-Ramos, et al. (1997). "Randomized trial of two doses of the prostaglandin E1 analog misoprostol for labor induction." Am J Obstet Gynecol **177**(2): 364-369; discussion 369-371.

Faundes, A., L. C. Santos, et al. (1996). "Post-abortion complications after interruption of pregnancy with misoprostol." Adv Contracept **12**(1): 1-9.

Fawole, A. O., O. S. Sotiloye, et al. (2011). "A double-blind, randomized, placebo-controlled trial of misoprostol and routine uterotonics for the prevention of postpartum hemorrhage." Int J Gynaecol Obstet **112**(2): 107-111.

Fawzy, M. and S. Abdel-Hady el (2010). "Midtrimester abortion using vaginal misoprostol for women with three or more prior cesarean deliveries." Int J Gynaecol Obstet **110**(1): 50-52.

Fekih, M., A. Jnifene, et al. (2009). "[Benefit of misoprostol for prevention of postpartum hemorrhage in cesarean section: a randomized controlled trial]." J Gynecol Obstet Biol Reprod (Paris) **38**(7): 588-593.

Feldman, D. M., A. F. Borgida, et al. (2003). "A randomized comparison of two regimens of misoprostol for second-trimester pregnancy termination." Am J Obstet Gynecol **189**(3): 710-713.

Ferguson, J. E., 2nd, B. H. Head, et al. (2002). "Misoprostol versus low-dose oxytocin for cervical ripening: a prospective, randomized, double-masked trial." Am J Obstet Gynecol **187**(2): 273-279; discussion 279-280.

Fiala, C., A. Aronsson, et al. (2005). "Effects of slow release misoprostol on uterine contractility in early pregnancy." Hum Reprod **20**(9): 2648-2652.

Ficicioglu, C., M. Tasdemir, et al. (1996). "Effect of vaginal misoprostol application for cervical softening in pregnancy interruption before ten weeks of gestation." Acta Obstet Gynecol Scand **75**(1): 54-56.

Filippini, A., G. Villa, et al. (2007). "Acute hemolytic anemia with acanthocytosis associated with high-dose misoprostol for medical abortion." Ann Emerg Med **50**(3): 289-291.

Fisher, S. A., V. P. Mackenzie, et al. (2001). "Oral versus vaginal misoprostol for induction of labor: a double-blind randomized controlled trial." Am J Obstet Gynecol **185**(4): 906-910.

Fittkow, C. T., H. Maul, et al. (2005). "Light-induced fluorescence of the human cervix decreases after prostaglandin application for induction of labor at term." Eur J Obstet Gynecol Reprod Biol **123**(1): 62-66.

Fletcher, H. and S. Hutchinson (2001). "A retrospective review of pregnancy outcome after misoprostol (prostaglandin E1) induction of labour." West Indian Med J **50**(1): 47-49.

Fletcher, H., S. Mitchell, et al. (1994). "Intravaginal misoprostol versus dinoprostone as cervical ripening and labor-inducing agents." Obstet Gynecol **83**(2): 244-247.

Fletcher, H. M., S. Mitchell, et al. (1993). "Intravaginal misoprostol as a cervical ripening agent." Br J Obstet Gynaecol **100**(7): 641-644.

Fong, Y. F., K. Singh, et al. (1998). "A comparative study using two dose regimens (200 microg or 400 microg) of vaginal misoprostol for pre-operative cervical dilatation in first trimester nulliparae." Br J Obstet Gynaecol **105**(4): 413-417.

Fong, Y. F., K. Singh, et al. (1999). "Severe hyperthermia following use of vaginal misoprostol for pre-operative cervical priming." Int J Gynaecol Obstet **64**(1): 73-74.

Fonseca, L., H. C. Wood, et al. (2008). "Randomized trial of preinduction cervical ripening: misoprostol vs oxytocin." Am J Obstet Gynecol **199**(3): 305 e301-305.

Fonseca, W., A. J. Alencar, et al. (1993). "Congenital malformation of the scalp and cranium after failed first trimester abortion attempt with misoprostol." Clin Dysmorphol **2**(1): 76-80.

Fontanarosa, M., S. Galiberti, et al. (2007). "Fertility after non-surgical management of the symptomatic first-trimester spontaneous abortion." Minerva Ginecol **59**(6): 591-594.

Frohn, W. E., S. Simmons, et al. (2002). "Prostaglandin E2 gel versus misoprostol for cervical ripening in patients with premature rupture of membranes after 34 weeks." Obstet Gynecol **99**(2): 206-210.

Gaffaney, C. A., L. L. Saul, et al. (2009). "Outpatient oral misoprostol for prolonged pregnancies: a pilot investigation." Am J Perinatol **26**(9): 673-677.

Gagne, A., E. Guilbert, et al. (2010). "Assessment of pain after elective abortion relating to the use of misoprostol for dilatation of the cervix." J Obstet Gynaecol Can **32**(3): 244-253.

Ganguly, R. P., S. P. Saha, et al. (2010). "A comparative study on sublingual versus oral and vaginal administration of misoprostol for late first and early second trimester abortion." J Indian Med Assoc **108**(5): 283-284, 286.

Gardeil, F., G. Gaffney, et al. (2001). "Severe HELLP syndrome remote from term." Ir Med J **94**(2): 54.

Garg, P., S. Batra, et al. (2005). "Oral misoprostol versus injectable methylergometrine in management of the third stage of labor." Int J Gynaecol Obstet **91**(2): 160-161.

Garry, D., R. Figueroa, et al. (2003). "Randomized controlled trial of vaginal misoprostol versus dinoprostone vaginal insert for labor induction." J Matern Fetal Neonatal Med **13**(4): 254-259.

Gelisen, O., E. Caliskan, et al. (2005). "Induction of labor with three different techniques at 41 weeks of gestation or spontaneous follow-up until 42 weeks in women with definitely unfavorable cervical scores." Eur J Obstet Gynecol Reprod Biol **120**(2): 164-169.

Geller, S. E., S. S. Goudar, et al. (2008). "Factors associated with acute postpartum hemorrhage in low-risk women delivering in rural India." Int J Gynaecol Obstet **101**(1): 94-99.

Gerstenfeld, T. S. and D. A. Wing (2001). "Rectal misoprostol versus intravenous oxytocin for the prevention of postpartum hemorrhage after vaginal delivery." <u>Am J Obstet Gynecol</u> **185**(4): 878-882.

Gherman, R. B., J. Browning, et al. (2001). "Oral misoprostol vs. intravaginal prostaglandin E2 for preinduction cervical ripening. A randomized trial." <u>J Reprod Med</u> **46**(7): 641-646.

Ghorab, M. N. and B. A. El Helw (1998). "Second-trimester termination of pregnancy by extra-amniotic prostaglandin F2alpha or endocervical misoprostol. A comparative study." <u>Acta Obstet Gynecol Scand</u> **77**(4): 429-432.

Gilbert, A. and R. Reid (2001). "A randomised trial of oral versus vaginal administration of misoprostol for the purpose of mid-trimester termination of pregnancy." <u>Aust N Z J Obstet Gynaecol</u> **41**(4): 407-410.

Gilles, J. M., M. D. Creinin, et al. (2004). "A randomized trial of saline solution-moistened misoprostol versus dry misoprostol for first-trimester pregnancy failure." <u>Am J Obstet Gynecol</u> **190**(2): 389-394.

Goldberg, A. B., E. A. Drey, et al. (2005). "Misoprostol compared with laminaria before early second-trimester surgical abortion: a randomized trial." <u>Obstet Gynecol</u> **106**(2): 234-241.

Gonzalez, C. H., M. J. Marques-Dias, et al. (1998). "Congenital abnormalities in Brazilian children associated with misoprostol misuse in first trimester of pregnancy." <u>Lancet</u> **351**(9116): 1624-1627.

Gonzalez, C. H., F. R. Vargas, et al. (1993). "Limb deficiency with or without Mobius sequence in seven Brazilian children associated with misoprostol use in the first trimester of pregnancy." <u>Am J Med Genet</u> **47**(1): 59-64.

Gonzalez, J. A., S. J. Carlan, et al. (2001). "Outpatient second trimester pregnancy termination." <u>Contraception</u> **63**(2): 89-93.

Gottschall, D. S., A. F. Borgida, et al. (1997). "A randomized clinical trial comparing misoprostol with prostaglandin E2 gel for preinduction cervical ripening." <u>Am J Obstet Gynecol</u> **177**(5): 1067-1070.

Grapsas, X., V. Liberis, et al. (2008). "Misoprostol and first trimester pregnancy termination." Clin Exp Obstet Gynecol **35**(1): 32-34.

Graziosi, G. C., B. W. Mol, et al. (2004). "Misoprostol versus curettage in women with early pregnancy failure after initial expectant management: a randomized trial." Hum Reprod **19**(8): 1894-1899.

Green, J., L. Borgatta, et al. (2007). "Intervention rates for placental removal following induction abortion with misoprostol." Contraception **76**(4): 310-313.

Greybush, M., C. Singleton, et al. (2001). "Preinduction cervical ripening techniques compared." J Reprod Med **46**(1): 11-17.

Gribel, G. P., L. G. Coca-Velarde, et al. (2010). "Electroacupuncture for cervical ripening prior to labor induction: a randomized clinical trial." Arch Gynecol Obstet.

Gronlund, L., A. L. Gronlund, et al. (2002). "Spontaneous abortion: expectant management, medical treatment or surgical evacuation." Acta Obstet Gynecol Scand **81**(8): 781-782.

Guix, C., M. Palacio, et al. (2005). "Efficacy of two regimens of misoprostol for early second-trimester pregnancy termination." Fetal Diagn Ther **20**(6): 544-548.

Gulmezoglu, A. M., J. Villar, et al. (2001). "WHO multicentre randomised trial of misoprostol in the management of the third stage of labour." Lancet **358**(9283): 689-695.

Gunalp, S. and I. Bildirici (2000). "The effect of vaginal pH on the efficacy of vaginal misoprostol for induction of labor." Acta Obstet Gynecol Scand **79**(4): 283-285.

Haberal, A., H. Celikkanat, et al. (1996). "Oral misoprostol use in early complicated pregnancy." Adv Contracept **12**(2): 139-143.

Hackney, D. N., M. D. Creinin, et al. (2007). "Medical management of early pregnancy failure in a patient with coronary artery disease." Fertil Steril **88**(1): 212 e211-213.

Hall, R., M. Duarte-Gardea, et al. (2002). "Oral versus vaginal misoprostol for labor induction." Obstet Gynecol **99**(6): 1044-1048.

Hamm, J., Z. Russell, et al. (2005). "Buccal misoprostol to prevent hemorrhage at cesarean delivery: a randomized study." Am J Obstet Gynecol **192**(5): 1404-1406.

Hamoda, H., P. W. Ashok, et al. (2004). "A randomized controlled comparison of sublingual and vaginal administration of misoprostol for cervical priming before first-trimester surgical abortion." Am J Obstet Gynecol **190**(1): 55-59.

Haque, N., L. Bilkis, et al. (2009). "Comparative study between rectally administered misoprostol as a prophylaxis versus conventional intramuscular oxytocin in post partum hemorrhage." Mymensingh Med J **18**(1 Suppl): S40-44.

Harriott, J., L. Christie, et al. (2009). "A randomized comparison of rectal misoprostol with syntometrine on blood loss in the third stage of labour." West Indian Med J **58**(3): 201-206.

Has, R., C. Batukan, et al. (2002). "Comparison of 25 and 50 microg vaginally administered misoprostol for preinduction of cervical ripening and labor induction." Gynecol Obstet Invest **53**(1): 16-21.

Hascalik, S., O. Celik, et al. (2005). "Influence of misoprostol (PGE1) on amniotic fluid and maternal serum adrenomedullin levels." Acta Obstet Gynecol Scand **84**(9): 833-836.

Henriques, A., A. V. Lourenco, et al. (2007). "Maternal death related to misoprostol overdose." Obstet Gynecol **109**(2 Pt2): 489-490.

Henry, A. M. and M. Haukkamaa (1999). "Comparison of vaginal misoprostol and gemeprost as pre-treatment in first trimester pregnancy interruption." Br J Obstet Gynaecol **106**(6): 540-543.

Herabutya, Y., B. Chanarachakul, et al. (2003). "Induction of labor with vaginal misoprostol for second trimester termination of pregnancy in the scarred uterus." Int J Gynaecol Obstet **83**(3): 293-297.

Herabutya, Y., B. Chanrachakul, et al. (2000). "Vaginal misoprostol in termination of second trimester pregnancy." J Obstet Gynaecol Res **26**(2): 121-125.

Herabutya, Y., B. Chanrachakul, et al. (2001). "Second trimester pregnancy termination: a comparison of 600 and 800 micrograms of intravaginal misoprostol." J Obstet Gynaecol Res **27**(3): 125-128.

Herabutya, Y., B. Chanrachakul, et al. (2005). "A randomised controlled trial of 6 and 12 hourly administration of vaginal misoprostol for second trimester pregnancy termination." BJOG **112**(9): 1297-1301.

Herabutya, Y. and O. P. P (1997). "Misoprostol in the management of missed abortion." Int J Gynaecol Obstet **56**(3): 263-266.

Herabutya, Y. and O. P. P (1998). "Second trimester abortion using intravaginal misoprostol." Int J Gynaecol Obstet **60**(2): 161-165.

Herabutya, Y., O. P. P, et al. (1997). "A comparison of intravaginal misoprostol and intracervical prostaglandin E2 gel for ripening of unfavorable cervix and labor induction." J Obstet Gynaecol Res **23**(4): 369-374.

Hern, W. M. (2001). "Laminaria, induced fetal demise and misoprostol in late abortion." Int J Gynaecol Obstet **75**(3): 279-286.

Hern, W. M. (2005). "Misoprostol as an adjunctive medication in late surgical abortion." Int J Gynaecol Obstet **88**(3): 327-328.

Hidar, S., M. Bouddebous, et al. (2005). "Randomized controlled trial of vaginal misoprostol versus vaginal misoprostol and isosorbide dinitrate for termination of pregnancy at 13-29 weeks." Arch Gynecol Obstet **273**(3): 157-160.

Hidar, S., M. Fekih, et al. (2001). "[Oxytocin and misoprostol administered intravaginally for termination of pregnancy at 13 to 29 weeks of amenorrhea. A prospective randomized trial]." J Gynecol Obstet Biol Reprod (Paris) **30**(5): 439-443.

Hill, D. A., R. A. Chez, et al. (2000). "Uterine rupture and dehiscence associated with intravaginal misoprostol cervical ripening." J Reprod Med **45**(10): 823-826.

Hill, J. B., B. D. Thigpen, et al. (2009). "A randomized clinical trial comparing vaginal misoprostol versus cervical Foley plus oral misoprostol for cervical ripening and labor induction." Am J Perinatol **26**(1): 33-38.

Ho, V., S. Keating, et al. (2007). "Misoprostol associated refractile material in fetal and placental tissues after medical termination of pregnancy." Am J Surg Pathol **31**(12): 1893-1896.

Hoffman, M. K. and A. C. Sciscione (2004). "Placenta accreta and intrauterine fetal death in a woman with prior endometrial ablation: a case report." J Reprod Med **49**(5): 384-386.

Hoffmann, R. A., J. Anthony, et al. (2001). "Oral misoprostol vs. placebo in the management of prelabor rupture of membranes at term." Int J Gynaecol Obstet **72**(3): 215-221.

Hofmeyr, G. J., Z. Alfirevic, et al. (2001). "Titrated oral misoprostol solution for induction of labour: a multi-centre, randomised trial." BJOG **108**(9): 952-959.

Hofmeyr, G. J., B. Fawole, et al. "Administration of 400 mug of misoprostol to augment routine active management of the third stage of labor." Int J Gynaecol Obstet **112**(2): 98-102.

Hofmeyr, G. J., S. Ferreira, et al. (2004). "Misoprostol for treating postpartum haemorrhage: a randomized controlled trial [ISRCTN72263357]." BMC Pregnancy Childbirth **4**(1): 16.

Hofmeyr, G. J., B. B. Matonhodze, et al. (2001). "Titrated oral misoprostol solution--a new method of labour induction." S Afr Med J **91**(9): 775-776.

Hofmeyr, G. J., D. Milos, et al. (1998). "Limb reduction anomaly after failed misoprostol abortion." S Afr Med J **88**(5): 566-567.

Hofmeyr, G. J., V. C. Nikodem, et al. (2001). "Side-effects of oral misoprostol in the third stage of labour--a randomised placebo-controlled trial." S Afr Med J **91**(5): 432-435.

Hofmeyr, G. J., V. C. Nikodem, et al. (1998). "A randomised placebo controlled trial of oral misoprostol in the third stage of labour." Br J Obstet Gynaecol **105**(9): 971-975.

Hoj, L., P. Cardoso, et al. (2005). "Effect of sublingual misoprostol on severe postpartum haemorrhage in a primary health centre in Guinea-Bissau: randomised double blind clinical trial." BMJ **331**(7519): 723.

How, H. Y., L. Leaseburge, et al. (2001). "A comparison of various routes and dosages of misoprostol for cervical ripening and the induction of labor." Am J Obstet Gynecol **185**(4): 911-915.

Hsieh, Y. Y., H. D. Tsai, et al. (2000). "Precipitate delivery and postpartum hemorrhage after term induction with 200 micrograms misoprostol." Zhonghua Yi Xue Za Zhi (Taipei) **63**(1): 58-61.

Inal, M. M., K. Ertopcu, et al. (2003). "The effect of oral versus vaginal misoprostol on cervical dilatation in first-trimester abortion: a double-blind, randomized study." Eur J Contracept Reprod Health Care **8**(4): 197-202.

Incerpi, M. H., M. J. Fassett, et al. (2001). "Vaginally administered misoprostol for outpatient cervical ripening in pregnancies complicated by diabetes mellitus." Am J Obstet Gynecol **185**(4): 916-919.

Jabir, M. and R. I. Smeet (2009). "Comparison of oral and vaginal misoprostol for cervical ripening before evacuation of first trimester missed miscarriage." Saudi Med J **30**(1): 82-87.

Jain, J. K., B. Harwood, et al. (2001). "Early pregnancy termination with vaginal misoprostol combined with loperamide and acetaminophen prophylaxis." Contraception **63**(4): 217-221.

Jain, J. K., J. Kuo, et al. (1999). "A comparison of two dosing regimens of intravaginal misoprostol for second-trimester pregnancy termination." Obstet Gynecol **93**(4): 571-575.

Jain, J. K. and D. R. Mishell, Jr. (1994). "A comparison of intravaginal misoprostol with prostaglandin E2 for termination of second-trimester pregnancy." N Engl J Med **331**(5): 290-293.

Jain, J. K. and D. R. Mishell, Jr. (1996). "A comparison of misoprostol with and without laminaria tents for induction of second-trimester abortion." Am J Obstet Gynecol **175**(1): 173-177.

Jones, M. M. and K. Fraser (1998). "Misoprostol and attempted self-induction of abortion." J R Soc Med **91**(4): 204-205.

Kaponis, A., S. Papatheodorou, et al. (2010). "Septic shock due to Klebsiella pneumoniae after medical abortion with misoprostol-only regimen." Fertil Steril **94**(4): 1529 e1523-1525.

Kapp, N., C. S. Todd, et al. (2007). "A randomized comparison of misoprostol to intrauterine instillation of hypertonic saline plus a prostaglandin F2alpha analogue for second-trimester induction termination in Uzbekistan." Contraception **76**(6): 461-466.

Karkanis, S. G., D. Caloia, et al. (2002). "Randomized controlled trial of rectal misoprostol versus oxytocin in third stage management." J Obstet Gynaecol Can **24**(2): 149-154.

Karsidag, A. Y., E. E. Buyukbayrak, et al. (2009). "Vaginal versus sublingual misoprostol for second-trimester pregnancy termination and effect on Doppler measurements." Int J Gynaecol Obstet **106**(3): 250-253.

Kashanian, M., A. R. Akbarian, et al. (2006). "Cervical ripening and induction of labor with intravaginal misoprostol and Foley catheter cervical traction." Int J Gynaecol Obstet **92**(1): 79-80.

Katz, V. L., R. M. Farmer, et al. (2000). "Use of misoprostol for cervical ripening." South Med J **93**(9): 881-884.

Kelekci, S., E. Erdemoglu, et al. (2006). "Randomized study on the effect of adding oxytocin to ethacridine lactate or misoprostol for second-trimester termination of pregnancy." Acta Obstet Gynecol Scand **85**(7): 825-829.

Kelekci, S., B. Yilmaz, et al. (2004). "Misoprostol wetting with acetic acid for pre-abortion cervical priming." Int J Gynaecol Obstet **85**(2): 188-189.

Khazardoost, S., S. Hantoushzadeh, et al. (2007). "A randomised trial of two regimens of vaginal misoprostol to manage termination of pregnancy of up to 16 weeks." Aust N Z J Obstet Gynaecol **47**(3): 226-229.

Khoury, A. N., Q. P. Zhou, et al. (2001). "A comparison of intermittent vaginal administration of two different doses of misoprostol suppositories with continuous dinoprostone for cervical ripening and labor induction." J Matern Fetal Med **10**(3): 186-192.

Kimya, Y., K. Ozerkan, et al. (2004). "Dehydroepiandrosterone sulfate levels and success of labor induction." Int J Gynaecol Obstet **86**(1): 33-34.

Kipikasa, J. H., C. D. Adair, et al. (2005). "Use of misoprostol on an outpatient basis for postdate pregnancy." Int J Gynaecol Obstet **88**(2): 108-111.

Kochhar, P. K., G. Gandhi, et al. (2010). "Evaluation of intravaginal misoprostol for medical management of pregnancies less than 20 weeks of gestation with absent cardiac activity." J Obstet Gynaecol Res **36**(3): 626-633.

Koskas, M., M. Jerbi, et al. (2005). "[Operative termination of pregnancy between 12 and 14 weeks' gestation: influence of the operator's experience]." J Gynecol Obstet Biol Reprod (Paris) **34**(4): 334-338.

Kovavisarach, E. and C. Jamnansiri (2005). "Intravaginal misoprostol 600 microg and 800 microg for the treatment of early pregnancy failure." Int J Gynaecol Obstet **90**(3): 208-212.

Kovavisarach, E. and U. Sathapanachai (2002). "Intravaginal 400 microg misoprostol for pregnancy termination in cases of blighted ovum: a randomised controlled trial." Aust N Z J Obstet Gynaecol **42**(2): 161-163.

Krithika, K. S., N. Aggarwal, et al. (2008). "Prospective randomised controlled trial to compare safety and efficacy of intravaginal Misoprostol with intracervical Cerviprime for induction of labour with unfavourable cervix." J Obstet Gynaecol **28**(3): 294-297.

Kundodyiwa, T. W., F. Majoko, et al. (2001). "Misoprostol versus oxytocin in the third stage of labor." Int J Gynaecol Obstet **75**(3): 235-241.

Kunwar, S., P. K. Saha, et al. (2010). "Second trimester pregnancy termination with 400 mug vaginal misoprostol: efficacy and safety." Biosci Trends **4**(6): 351-354.

Kwon, J. S., G. A. Davies, et al. (2001). "A comparison of oral and vaginal misoprostol for induction of labour at term: a randomised trial." BJOG **108**(1): 23-26.

Lam, H., O. S. Tang, et al. (2004). "A pilot-randomized comparison of sublingual misoprostol with syntometrine on the blood loss in third stage of labor." Acta Obstet Gynecol Scand **83**(7): 647-650.

Lamina, M. A., B. O. Akinyemi, et al. (2005). "Abdominal pregnancy: a cause of failed induction of labour." Niger J Med **14**(2): 213-217.

Langenegger, E. J., H. J. Odendaal, et al. (2005). "Oral misoprostol versus intracervical dinoprostone for induction of labor." Int J Gynaecol Obstet **88**(3): 242-248.

Langer, B. R., C. Peter, et al. (2004). "Second and third medical termination of pregnancy with misoprostol without mifepristone." Fetal Diagn Ther **19**(3): 266-270.

Lapaire, O., M. C. Schneider, et al. (2006). "Oral misoprostol vs. intravenous oxytocin in reducing blood loss after emergency cesarean delivery." Int J Gynaecol Obstet **95**(1): 2-7.

Lawrie, A., G. Penney, et al. (1996). "A randomised comparison of oral and vaginal misoprostol for cervical priming before suction termination of pregnancy." Br J Obstet Gynaecol **103**(11): 1117-1119.

le Roux, P. A., J. O. Olarogun, et al. (2002). "Oral and vaginal misoprostol compared with dinoprostone for induction of labor: a randomized controlled trial." Obstet Gynecol **99**(2): 201-205.

Leader, J., M. Bujnovsky, et al. (2002). "Effect of oral misoprostol after second-trimester delivery: a randomized, blinded study." Obstet Gynecol **100**(4): 689-694.

Ledingham, M. A., A. J. Thomson, et al. (2001). "A comparison of isosorbide mononitrate, misoprostol and combination therapy for first trimester pre-operative cervical ripening: a randomised controlled trial." BJOG **108**(3): 276-280.

Lee, H. Y. (1997). "A randomised double-blind study of vaginal misoprostol vs dinoprostone for cervical ripening and labour induction in prolonged pregnancy." Singapore Med J **38**(7): 292-294.

Lee, V. C., E. H. Ng, et al. (2011). "Misoprostol with or without letrozole pretreatment for termination of pregnancy: a randomized controlled trial." Obstet Gynecol **117**(2 Pt 1): 317-323.

Leszczynska-Gorzelak, B., M. Laskowska, et al. (2001). "Comparative analysis of the effectiveness of misoprostol and prostaglandin E(2) in the preinduction and induction of labor." Med Sci Monit **7**(5): 1023-1028.

Levey, K. A., A. P. MacKenzie, et al. (2004). "Increased rates of chorioamnionitis with extra-amniotic saline infusion method of labor induction." Obstet Gynecol **103**(4): 724-728.

Levy, R., E. Vaisbuch, et al. (2007). "Induction of labor with oral misoprostol for premature rupture of membranes at term in women with unfavorable cervix: a randomized, double-blind, placebo-controlled trial." J Perinat Med **35**(2): 126-129.

Li, C. F., C. W. Chan, et al. (2003). "A comparison of isosorbide mononitrate and misoprostol cervical ripening before suction evacuation." Obstet Gynecol **102**(3): 583-588.

Li, C. F., C. W. Chan, et al. (2003). "A study of the efficacy of cervical ripening with nitric oxide donor versus placebo for cervical priming before second-trimester termination of pregnancy." Contraception **68**(4): 269-272.

Li, C. F., C. Y. Wong, et al. (2003). "A study of co-treatment of nonsteroidal anti-inflammatory drugs (NSAIDs) with misoprostol for cervical priming before suction termination of first trimester pregnancy." Contraception **67**(2): 101-105.

Li, Y. T., G. Q. Hou, et al. (2008). "High-dose misoprostol as an alternative therapy after failed medical abortion." Taiwan J Obstet Gynecol **47**(4): 408-411.

Li, Y. T. and C. S. Yin (2001). "Delivery of retained placenta by misoprostol in second trimester abortion." Int J Gynaecol Obstet **74**(2): 215-216.

Lialios, G., A. Kallitsaris, et al. (2006). "Uterine perforation as a rare complication of attempted pregnancy termination with misoprostol: a case report." J Reprod Med **51**(7): 599-600.

Liaquat, N. F., I. Javed, et al. (2006). "Therapeutic termination of second trimester pregnancies with low dose misoprostol." J Coll Physicians Surg Pak **16**(7): 464-467.

Lim, J. M., E. B. Soh, et al. (1995). "Intravaginal misoprostol for termination of midtrimester pregnancy." Aust N Z J Obstet Gynaecol **35**(1): 54-55.

Liu, H. S., T. Y. Chu, et al. (1999). "Intracervical misoprostol as an effective method of labor induction at term." Int J Gynaecol Obstet **64**(1): 49-53.

Lo, J. Y., J. M. Alexander, et al. (2003). "Ruptured membranes at term: randomized, double-blind trial of oral misoprostol for labor induction." Obstet Gynecol **101**(4): 685-689.

Lo, T. K., W. L. Lau, et al. (2008). "The effect of gestational age on the outcome of second-trimester termination of pregnancies for foetal abnormalities." Prenat Diagn **28**(6): 508-511.

Lo, T. K., W. L. Lau, et al. (2008). "Effect of fetal diagnosis on the outcomes of second-trimester pregnancy termination for fetal abnormalities: a pilot study." J Matern Fetal Neonatal Med **21**(8): 523-527.

Lo, T. K., W. L. Lau, et al. (2008). "Association between lethal fetal anomalies and lower risk for incomplete medical termination of pregnancy." Int J Gynaecol Obstet **102**(2): 176-178.

Lokugamage, A. U., S. F. Forsyth, et al. (2003). "Dinoprostone versus misoprostol: a randomized study of nulliparous women undergoing induction of labor." Acta Obstet Gynecol Scand **82**(2): 133-137.

Lokugamage, A. U., S. F. Forsyth, et al. (2003). "Randomized trial in multiparous patients: investigating a single vs. two-dose regimen of intravaginal misoprostol for induction of labor." Acta Obstet Gynecol Scand **82**(2): 138-142.

Lokugamage, A. U., M. Paine, et al. (2001). "Active management of the third stage at caesarean section: a randomised controlled trial of misoprostol versus syntocinon." Aust N Z J Obstet Gynaecol **41**(4): 411-414.

Lokugamage, A. U., K. R. Sullivan, et al. (2001). "A randomized study comparing rectally administered misoprostol versus Syntometrine combined with an oxytocin infusion for the cessation of primary post partum hemorrhage." Acta Obstet Gynecol Scand **80**(9): 835-839.

Low, Y. S., T. Adams, et al. (2009). "Uterine rupture during the mid-trimester management of intrauterine fetal death." J Obstet Gynaecol **29**(5): 443.

Lumbiganon, P., J. Villar, et al. (2002). "Side effects of oral misoprostol during the first 24 hours after administration in the third stage of labour." BJOG **109**(11): 1222-1226.

Machtinger, R., D. Stockheim, et al. (2009). "Medical treatment with misoprostol for early failure of pregnancies after assisted reproductive technology: a promising treatment option." Fertil Steril **91**(5): 1881-1885.

MacIsaac, L., D. Grossman, et al. (1999). "A randomized controlled trial of laminaria, oral misoprostol, and vaginal misoprostol before abortion." Obstet Gynecol **93**(5 Pt 1): 766-770.

Magtibay, P. M., K. D. Ramin, et al. (1998). "Misoprostol as a labor induction agent." J Matern Fetal Med **7**(1): 15-18.

Mahjabeen, N. P. Khawaja, et al. (2009). "Comparison of oral versus vaginal misoprostol for mid-trimester pregnancy termination." J Coll Physicians Surg Pak **19**(6): 359-362.

Mahlmeister, L. (2005). "Best practices in perinatal and neonatal nursing: cervical ripeners and the induction of labor." J Perinat Neonatal Nurs **19**(2): 97-99.

Majoko, F., T. Magwali, et al. (2002). "Uterine rupture associated with use of misoprostol for induction of labor." Int J Gynaecol Obstet **76**(1): 77-78.

Majoko, F., L. Nystrom, et al. (2002). "No benefit, but increased harm from high dose (100 microg) misoprostol for induction of labour: a randomised trial of high vs. low (50 microg) dose misoprostol." J Obstet Gynaecol **22**(6): 614-617.

Majoko, F., M. Zwizwai, et al. (2002). "Labor induction with vaginal misoprostol and extra-amniotic prostaglandin F2alpha gel." Int J Gynaecol Obstet **76**(2): 127-133.

Majoko, F., M. Zwizwai, et al. (2002). "Vaginal misoprostol for induction of labour: a more effective agent than prostaglandin F2 alpha gel and prostaglandin E2 pessary." Cent Afr J Med **48**(11-12): 123-128.

Makhlouf, A. M., T. K. Al-Hussaini, et al. (2003). "Second-trimester pregnancy termination: comparison of three different methods." J Obstet Gynaecol **23**(4): 407-411.

Malapati, R., G. Villaluna, et al. (2011). "Use of misoprostol for pregnancy termination in women with prior classical cesarean delivery: a report of 3 cases." J Reprod Med **56**(1-2): 85-86.

Mansouri, H. A. and N. Alsahly (2010). "Rectal versus oral misoprostol for active management of third stage of labor: a randomized controlled trial." Arch Gynecol Obstet.

Mao, S. P., C. C. Chang, et al. (2007). "Gestational thrombocytopenia complicated with macrosomia, failure to progress in active labor, and postpartum hemorrhage." Taiwan J Obstet Gynecol **46**(2): 177-179.

Marques-Dias, M. J., C. H. Gonzalez, et al. (2003). "Mobius sequence in children exposed in utero to misoprostol: neuropathological study of three cases." Birth Defects Res A Clin Mol Teratol **67**(12): 1002-1007.

Marquette, G. P., M. A. Skoll, et al. (2005). "A randomized trial comparing oral misoprostol with intra-amniotic prostaglandin F2alpha for second trimester terminations." J Obstet Gynaecol Can **27**(11): 1013-1018.

Martinez de Tejada, B., G. Martillotti, et al. (2010). "The risk of placental abruption when using prostaglandins for cervical ripening in women with preeclampsia: comparing misoprostol versus dinoprostone." J Matern Fetal Neonatal Med **23**(9): 988-993.

Matonhodze, B. B., G. J. Hofmeyr, et al. (2003). "Labour induction at term--a randomised trial comparing Foley catheter plus titrated oral misoprostol solution, titrated oral misoprostol solution alone, and dinoprostone." S Afr Med J **93**(5): 375-379.

Mazzone, M. E. and J. Woolever (2006). "Uterine rupture in a patient with an unscarred uterus: a case study." WMJ **105**(2): 64-66.

McKenna, D. S., J. B. Ester, et al. (2004). "Misoprostol outpatient cervical ripening without subsequent induction of labor: a randomized trial." Obstet Gynecol **104**(3): 579-584.

Megalo, A., P. Petignat, et al. (2004). "Influence of misoprostol or prostaglandin E(2) for induction of labor on the incidence of pathological CTG tracing: a randomized trial." Eur J Obstet Gynecol Reprod Biol **116**(1): 34-38.

Menakaya, U., V. Otoide, et al. (2005). "Experience with misoprostol in the management of missed abortion in the second trimester." J Obstet Gynaecol **25**(6): 583-585.

Mendilcioglu, I., M. Simsek, et al. (2002). "Misoprostol in second and early third trimester for termination of pregnancies with fetal anomalies." Int J Gynaecol Obstet **79**(2): 131-135.

Meydanli, M. M., E. Caliskan, et al. (2003). "Labor induction post-term with 25 micrograms vs. 50 micrograms of intravaginal misoprostol." Int J Gynaecol Obstet **81**(3): 249-255.

Meyer, M., J. Pflum, et al. (2005). "Outpatient misoprostol compared with dinoprostone gel for preinduction cervical ripening: a randomized controlled trial." Obstet Gynecol **105**(3): 466-472.

Miller, S., C. Tudor, et al. (2009). "Randomized double masked trial of Zhi Byed 11, a Tibetan traditional medicine, versus misoprostol to prevent postpartum hemorrhage in Lhasa, Tibet." J Midwifery Womens Health **54**(2): 133-141 e131.

Mirmilstein, V., S. Rowlands, et al. (2009). "Outcomes for subsequent pregnancy in women who have undergone misoprostol mid-trimester termination of pregnancy." Aust N Z J Obstet Gynaecol **49**(2): 195-197.

Mittal, S., R. Sehgal, et al. (2011). "Cervical priming with misoprostol before manual vacuum aspiration versus electric vacuum aspiration for first-trimester surgical abortion." Int J Gynaecol Obstet **112**(1): 34-39.

Mobeen, N., J. Durocher, et al. (2011). "Administration of misoprostol by trained traditional birth attendants to prevent postpartum haemorrhage in homebirths in Pakistan: a randomised placebo-controlled trial." BJOG **118**(3): 353-361.

Moodley, J., S. Venkatachalam, et al. (2003). "Misoprostol for cervical ripening at and near term--a comparative study." S Afr Med J **93**(5): 371-374.

Moodliar, S., J. S. Bagratee, et al. (2005). "Medical vs. surgical evacuation of first-trimester spontaneous abortion." Int J Gynaecol Obstet **91**(1): 21-26.

Moraes Filho, O. B., R. M. Albuquerque, et al. (2010). "A randomized controlled trial comparing vaginal misoprostol versus Foley catheter plus oxytocin for labor induction." Acta Obstet Gynecol Scand **89**(8): 1045-1052.

Moreno-Ruiz, N. L., J. L. Vesona, et al. (2009). "Misoprostol priming prior to second trimester medical abortion." Int J Gynaecol Obstet **106**(1): 67-68.

Mostafa-Gharebaghi, P., M. Mansourfar, et al. (2010). "Low dose vaginal misoprostol versus prostaglandin E2 suppository for early uterine evacuation: a randomized clinical trial." Pak J Biol Sci **13**(19): 946-950.

Mousavi, S. A. and F. Behnamfar (2009). "Gestational trophoblastic tumor with liver metastasis after misoprostol abortion." Arch Gynecol Obstet **279**(4): 587-590.

Mozurkewich, E., J. Horrocks, et al. (2003). "The MisoPROM study: a multicenter randomized comparison of oral misoprostol and oxytocin for premature rupture of membranes at term." Am J Obstet Gynecol **189**(4): 1026-1030.

Muffley, P. E., M. L. Stitely, et al. (2002). "Early intrauterine pregnancy failure: a randomized trial of medical versus surgical treatment." Am J Obstet Gynecol **187**(2): 321-325; discussion 325-326.

Mulayim, B., N. Y. Celik, et al. (2009). "Sublingual misoprostol after surgical management of early termination of pregnancy." Fertil Steril **92**(2): 678-681.

Mullin, P. M., M. House, et al. (2002). "A comparison of vaginally administered misoprostol with extra-amniotic saline solution infusion for cervical ripening and labor induction." Am J Obstet Gynecol **187**(4): 847-852.

Munthali, J. and J. Moodley (2001). "The use of misoprostol for mid-trimester therapeutic termination of pregnancy." Trop Doct **31**(3): 157-161.

Murchison, A. and P. Duff (2004). "Misoprostol for uterine evacuation in patients with early pregnancy failures." Am J Obstet Gynecol **190**(5): 1445-1446.

Naguib, A. H., H. M. Morsi, et al. (2010). "Vaginal misoprostol for second-trimester pregnancy termination after one previous cesarean delivery." Int J Gynaecol Obstet **108**(1): 48-51.

Nansel, T. R., F. Doyle, et al. (2005). "Quality of life in women undergoing medical treatment for early pregnancy failure." J Obstet Gynecol Neonatal Nurs **34**(4): 473-481.

Nasr, A., A. Y. Shahin, et al. (2009). "Rectal misoprostol versus intravenous oxytocin for prevention of postpartum hemorrhage." Int J Gynaecol Obstet **105**(3): 244-247.

Nayki, U., C. E. Taner, et al. (2005). "Uterine rupture during second trimester abortion with misoprostol." Fetal Diagn Ther **20**(5): 469-471.

Naz, S. and N. Sultana (2007). "Role of misoprostol for therapeutic termination of pregnancy from 10 -28 weeks of gestation." J Pak Med Assoc **57**(3): 129-132.

Neiger, R. and P. C. Greaves (2001). "Comparison between vaginal misoprostol and cervical dinoprostone for cervical ripening and labor induction." Tenn Med **94**(1): 25-27.

Nellore, V., S. Mittal, et al. (2006). "Rectal misoprostol vs. 15-methyl prostaglandin F2alpha for the prevention of postpartum hemorrhage." Int J Gynaecol Obstet **94**(1): 45-46.

Ng, P. S., A. S. Chan, et al. (2001). "A multicentre randomized controlled trial of oral misoprostol and i.m. syntometrine in the management of the third stage of labour." Hum Reprod **16**(1): 31-35.

Ng, P. S., C. Y. Lai, et al. (2007). "A double-blind randomized controlled trial of oral misoprostol and intramuscular syntometrine in the management of the third stage of labor." Gynecol Obstet Invest **63**(1): 55-60.

Ngai, S. W., Y. M. Chan, et al. (2000). "Labour characteristics and uterine activity: misoprostol compared with oxytocin in women at term with prelabour rupture of the membranes." BJOG **107**(2): 222-227.

Ngai, S. W., Y. M. Chan, et al. (1999). "The use of misoprostol for pre-operative cervical dilatation prior to vacuum aspiration: a randomized trial." Hum Reprod **14**(8): 2139-2142.

Ngai, S. W., Y. M. Chan, et al. (2001). "Vaginal misoprostol as medical treatment for first trimester spontaneous miscarriage." Hum Reprod **16**(7): 1493-1496.

Ngai, S. W., O. S. Tang, et al. (2000). "Vaginal misoprostol alone for medical abortion up to 9 weeks of gestation: efficacy and acceptability." Hum Reprod **15**(5): 1159-1162.

Ngai, S. W., O. S. Tang, et al. (1995). "Oral misoprostol versus placebo for cervical dilatation before vacuum aspiration in first trimester pregnancy." Hum Reprod **10**(5): 1220-1222.

Ngai, S. W., W. K. To, et al. (1996). "Cervical priming with oral misoprostol in pre-labor rupture of membranes at term." Obstet Gynecol **87**(6): 923-926.

Ngai, S. W., K. C. Yeung, et al. (1995). "Oral misoprostol versus vaginal gemeprost for cervical dilatation prior to vacuum aspiration in women in the sixth to twelfth week of gestation." Contraception **51**(6): 347-350.

Ngoc, N. T., J. Blum, et al. (2004). "Medical treatment of missed abortion using misoprostol." Int J Gynaecol Obstet **87**(2): 138-142.

Nguyen, T. N., J. Blum, et al. (2005). "A randomized controlled study comparing 600 versus 1,200 microg oral misoprostol for medical management of incomplete abortion." Contraception **72**(6): 438-442.

Nicholson, J. M., P. Cronholm, et al. (2009). "The association between increased use of labor induction and reduced rate of cesarean delivery." J Womens Health (Larchmt) **18**(11): 1747-1758.

Nigam, A., M. Madan, et al. (2010). "Labour induction with 25 micrograms versus 50 micrograms intravaginal misoprostol in full term pregnancies." Trop Doct **40**(1): 53-55.

Nigam, A., V. K. Singh, et al. (2004). "Misoprostol vs. oxytocin for induction of labor at term." Int J Gynaecol Obstet **86**(3): 398-400.

Nigam, A., V. K. Singh, et al. (2006). "Vaginal vs. oral misoprostol for mid-trimester abortion." Int J Gynaecol Obstet **92**(3): 270-271.

Niromanesh, S., M. Hashemi-Fesharaki, et al. (2005). "Second trimester abortion using intravaginal misoprostol." Int J Gynaecol Obstet **89**(3): 276-277.

Nor Azlin, M. I., H. S. Abdullah, et al. (2006). "Misoprostol (alone) in second trimester terminations of pregnancy: as effective as Gemeprost?" J Obstet Gynaecol **26**(6): 546-549.

Nucatola, D., N. Roth, et al. (2008). "Serious adverse events associated with the use of misoprostol alone for cervical preparation prior to early second trimester surgical abortion (12-16 weeks)." Contraception **78**(3): 245-248.

Nunes, F., R. Rodrigues, et al. (1999). "Randomized comparison between intravaginal misoprostol and dinoprostone for cervical ripening and induction of labor." <u>Am J Obstet Gynecol</u> **181**(3): 626-629.

Nuthalapaty, F. S., P. S. Ramsey, et al. (2005). "High-dose vaginal misoprostol versus concentrated oxytocin plus low-dose vaginal misoprostol for midtrimester labor induction: a randomized trial." <u>Am J Obstet Gynecol</u> **193**(3 Pt 2): 1065-1070.

Nuutila, M., J. Toivonen, et al. (1997). "A comparison between two doses of intravaginal misoprostol and gemeprost for induction of second-trimester abortion." <u>Obstet Gynecol</u> **90**(6): 896-900.

O'Brien, P., H. El-Refaey, et al. (1998). "Rectally administered misoprostol for the treatment of postpartum hemorrhage unresponsive to oxytocin and ergometrine: a descriptive study." <u>Obstet Gynecol</u> **92**(2): 212-214.

Oboro, V. O., A. I. Isawumi, et al. (2007). "Factors predicting failure of labour induction." <u>Niger Postgrad Med J</u> **14**(2): 137-139.

Oboro, V. O. and T. O. Tabowei (2003). "A randomised controlled trial of misoprostol versus oxytocin in the active management of the third stage of labour." <u>J Obstet Gynaecol</u> **23**(1): 13-16.

Oboro, V. O. and T. O. Tabowei (2005). "Outpatient misoprostol cervical ripening without subsequent induction of labor to prevent post-term pregnancy." <u>Acta Obstet Gynecol Scand</u> **84**(7): 628-631.

Oboro, V. O., T. O. Tabowei, et al. (2003). "Intrauterine misoprostol for refractory postpartum hemorrhage." <u>Int J Gynaecol Obstet</u> **80**(1): 67-68.

Odeh, M., R. Tendler, et al. (2010). "Early pregnancy failure: factors affecting successful medical treatment." <u>Isr Med Assoc J</u> **12**(6): 325-328.

Okanlomo, K. A., D. Ngotho, et al. (1999). "Effect of misoprostol for cervical ripening prior to pregnancy interruption before twelve weeks of gestation." <u>East Afr Med J</u> **76**(10): 552-555.

Okman-Kilic, T. and M. Kucuk (2004). "Rectal misoprostol vs vaginal misoprostol for first trimester termination of pregnancy." <u>Int J Gynaecol Obstet</u> **85**(1): 64-65.

Omole-Ohonsi, A., A. Ashimi, et al. (2009). "Spontaneous pre-labour rupture of membranes at term: immediate versus delayed induction of labour." West Afr J Med **28**(3): 156-160.

Oppegaard, K. S., M. Abdelnoor, et al. (2004). "The use of oral misoprostol for pre-abortion cervical priming: a randomised controlled trial of 400 versus 200 microg in first trimester pregnancies." BJOG **111**(2): 154-159.

Oppegaard, K. S., E. Qvigstad, et al. (2006). "Oral versus self-administered vaginal misoprostol at home before surgical termination of pregnancy: a randomised controlled trial." BJOG **113**(1): 58-64.

Orioli, I. M. and E. E. Castilla (2000). "Epidemiological assessment of misoprostol teratogenicity." BJOG **107**(4): 519-523.

Owen, J. and J. C. Hauth (1999). "Vaginal misoprostol vs. concentrated oxytocin plus low-dose prostaglandin E2 for second trimester pregnancy termination." J Matern Fetal Med **8**(2): 48-50.

Owolabi, A. T., O. Kuti, et al. (2005). "Randomised trial of intravaginal misoprostol and intracervical Foley catheter for cervical ripening and induction of labour." J Obstet Gynaecol **25**(6): 565-568.

Ozan, H., T. Bilgin, et al. (2000). "Misoprostol in uterine atony: a report of 2 cases." Clin Exp Obstet Gynecol **27**(3-4): 221-222.

Ozan, H., G. Uncu, et al. (2001). "Misoprostol in labor induction." J Obstet Gynaecol Res **27**(1): 17-20.

Ozden, S., M. N. Delikara, et al. (2002). "Intravaginal misoprostol vs. expectant management in premature rupture of membranes with low Bishop scores at term." Int J Gynaecol Obstet **77**(2): 109-115.

Ozerkan, K., G. Ocakoglu, et al. (2009). "A comparison of low-dose and high-dose protocols of vaginal misoprostol for second trimester termination of pregnancy." Clin Exp Obstet Gynecol **36**(4): 245-247.

Ozkaya, O., M. Sezik, et al. (2005). "Placebo-controlled randomized comparison of vaginal with rectal misoprostol in the prevention of postpartum hemorrhage." J Obstet Gynaecol Res **31**(5): 389-393.

Pacarada, M., F. Zeqiri, et al. (2011). "Misoprostol-induced abortions in Kosovo." Int J Gynaecol Obstet **112**(2): 116-118.

Panchal, H. B., E. M. Godfrey, et al. (2010). "Buccal misoprostol for cervical ripening prior to first trimester abortion." Contraception **81**(2): 161-164.

Pandian, Z., P. Ashok, et al. (2001). "The treatment of incomplete miscarriage with oral misoprostol." BJOG **108**(2): 213-214.

Pang, M. W., T. S. Lee, et al. (2001). "Incomplete miscarriage: a randomized controlled trial comparing oral with vaginal misoprostol for medical evacuation." Hum Reprod **16**(11): 2283-2287.

Paritakul, P. and V. Phupong (2010). "Comparative study between oral and sublingual 600 microg misoprostol for the treatment of incomplete abortion." J Obstet Gynaecol Res **36**(5): 978-983.

Patel, A., E. Talmont, et al. (2006). "Adequacy and safety of buccal misoprostol for cervical preparation prior to termination of second-trimester pregnancy." Contraception **73**(4): 420-430.

Patel, N., R. Shatzmiller, et al. (2008). "Cryptogenic stroke in the setting of intravaginal prostaglandin therapy for elective abortion." Clin Neurol Neurosurg **110**(5): 529-531.

Patted, S. S., S. S. Goudar, et al. (2009). "Side effects of oral misoprostol for the prevention of postpartum hemorrhage: results of a community-based randomised controlled trial in rural India." J Matern Fetal Neonatal Med **22**(1): 24-28.

Paungmora, N., Y. Herabutya, et al. (2004). "Comparison of oral and vaginal misoprostol for induction of labor at term: a randomized controlled trial." J Obstet Gynaecol Res **30**(5): 358-362.

Paz, B., G. Ohel, et al. (2002). "Second trimester abortion by laminaria followed by vaginal misoprostol or intrauterine prostaglandin F2alpha: a randomized trial." Contraception **65**(6): 411-413.

Perry, K. G., Jr., J. E. Larmon, et al. (1998). "Cervical ripening: a randomized comparison between intravaginal misoprostol and an intracervical balloon catheter combined with intravaginal dinoprostone." Am J Obstet Gynecol **178**(6): 1333-1340.

Perry, K. G., Jr., B. K. Rinehart, et al. (1999). "Second-trimester uterine evacuation: A comparison of intra-amniotic (15S)-15-methyl-prostaglandin F2alpha and intravaginal misoprostol." Am J Obstet Gynecol **181**(5 Pt 1): 1057-1061.

Pevzner, L., Z. Alfirevic, et al. (2011). "Cardiotocographic abnormalities associated with misoprostol and dinoprostone cervical ripening and labor induction." Eur J Obstet Gynecol Reprod Biol.

Pevzner, L., B. L. Powers, et al. (2009). "Effects of maternal obesity on duration and outcomes of prostaglandin cervical ripening and labor induction." Obstet Gynecol **114**(6): 1315-1321.

Pevzner, L., W. F. Rayburn, et al. (2009). "Factors predicting successful labor induction with dinoprostone and misoprostol vaginal inserts." Obstet Gynecol **114**(2 Pt 1): 261-267.

Phillip, H., H. Fletcher, et al. (2004). "The impact of induced labour on postpartum blood loss." J Obstet Gynaecol **24**(1): 12-15.

Phupong, V., S. Taneepanichskul, et al. (2004). "Comparative study between single dose 600 microg and repeated dose of oral misoprostol for treatment of incomplete abortion." Contraception **70**(4): 307-311.

Platz-Christensen, J. J., S. Nielsen, et al. (1995). "Is misoprostol the drug of choice for induced cervical ripening in early pregnancy termination?" Acta Obstet Gynecol Scand **74**(10): 809-812.

Politz, L. B., R. A. Chez, et al. (2001). "The effect of a pill inserter on vaginal misoprostol dosing." J Matern Fetal Med **10**(5): 332-334.

Pongsatha, S., N. Morakot, et al. (2002). "Demographic characteristics of women with self use of misoprostol for pregnancy interruption attending Maharaj Nakorn Chiang Mai Hospital." J Med Assoc Thai **85**(10): 1074-1080.

Pongsatha, S., S. Sirisukkasem, et al. (2002). "A comparison of 100 microg oral misoprostol every 3 hours and 6 hours for labor induction: a randomized controlled trial." J Obstet Gynaecol Res **28**(6): 308-312.

Pongsatha, S. and T. Tongsong (2001). "Second trimester pregnancy termination with 800 mcg vaginal misoprostol." J Med Assoc Thai **84**(6): 859-863.

Pongsatha, S. and T. Tongsong (2003). "Misoprostol for second trimester termination of pregnancies with prior low transverse cesarean section." Int J Gynaecol Obstet **80**(1): 61-62.

Pongsatha, S. and T. Tongsong (2004). "Intravaginal misoprostol for pregnancy termination." Int J Gynaecol Obstet **87**(2): 176-177.

Pongsatha, S. and T. Tongsong (2004). "Therapeutic termination of second trimester pregnancies with intrauterine fetal death with 400 micrograms of oral misoprostol." J Obstet Gynaecol Res **30**(3): 217-220.

Pongsatha, S. and T. Tongsong (2006). "Second-trimester pregnancy interruption with vaginal misoprostol in women with previous cesarean section." J Med Assoc Thai **89**(8): 1097-1100.

Pongsatha, S. and T. Tongsong (2008). "Randomized comparison of dry tablet insertion versus gel form of vaginal misoprostol for second trimester pregnancy termination." J Obstet Gynaecol Res **34**(2): 199-203.

Pongsatha, S., T. Tongsong, et al. (2001). "A comparison between 50 mcg oral misoprostol every 4 hours and 6 hours for labor induction: a prospective randomized controlled trial." J Med Assoc Thai **84**(7): 989-994.

Pongsatha, S., T. Tongsong, et al. (2001). "Therapeutic termination of second trimester pregnancy with vaginal misoprostol." J Med Assoc Thai **84**(4): 515-519.

Pongsatha, S., A. Vijittrawiwat, et al. (2005). "A comparison of labor induction by oral and vaginal misoprostol." Int J Gynaecol Obstet **88**(2): 140-141.

Poon, L. C. and J. Parsons (2007). "Audit of the effectiveness of cervical preparation with Dilapan prior to late second-trimester (20-24 weeks) surgical termination of pregnancy." BJOG **114**(4): 485-488.

Prachasilpchai, N., K. Russameecharoen, et al. (2006). "Success rate of second-trimester termination of pregnancy using misoprostol." J Med Assoc Thai **89**(8): 1115-1119.

Prasad, S., A. Kumar, et al. (2009). "Early termination of pregnancy by single-dose 800 microg misoprostol compared with surgical evacuation." Fertil Steril **91**(1): 28-31.

Prasartsakulchai, C. and Y. Tannirandorn (2004). "A comparison of vaginal misoprostol 800 microg versus 400 microg in early pregnancy failure: a randomized controlled trial." J Med Assoc Thai **87 Suppl 3**: S18-23.

Prata, N., A. Gessessew, et al. (2009). "Prevention of postpartum hemorrhage: options for home births in rural Ethiopia." Afr J Reprod Health **13**(2): 87-95.

Prata, N., S. Hamza, et al. (2006). "Misoprostol and active management of the third stage of labor." Int J Gynaecol Obstet **94**(2): 149-155.

Prata, N., G. Mbaruku, et al. (2005). "Controlling postpartum hemorrhage after home births in Tanzania." Int J Gynaecol Obstet **90**(1): 51-55.

Prata, N., G. Mbaruku, et al. (2009). "Community-based availability of misoprostol: is it safe?" Afr J Reprod Health **13**(2): 117-128.

Rabe, T., H. Basse, et al. (1987). "[Effect of the PGE1 methyl analog misoprostol on the pregnant uterus in the first trimester]." Geburtshilfe Frauenheilkd **47**(5): 324-331.

Radulovic, N., A. Norstrom, et al. (2007). "Outpatient cervical ripening before first-trimester surgical abortion: a comparison between misoprostol and isosorbide mononitrate." Acta Obstet Gynecol Scand **86**(3): 344-348.

Radulovic, N. V., E. Ekerhovd, et al. (2009). "Cervical priming in the first trimester: morphological and biochemical effects of misoprostol and isosorbide mononitrate." Acta Obstet Gynecol Scand **88**(1): 43-51.

Rae, D. W., F. W. Smith, et al. (2001). "Magnetic resonance imaging of the human cervix: a study of the effects of prostaglandins in the first trimester." Hum Reprod **16**(8): 1744-1747.

Raio, L., F. Ghezzi, et al. (2001). "[Shorter delivery time after induction with misoprostol]." Z Geburtshilfe Neonatol **205**(4): 147-151.

Rajbhandari, S., S. Hodgins, et al. (2010). "Expanding uterotonic protection following childbirth through community-based distribution of misoprostol: operations research study in Nepal." Int J Gynaecol Obstet **108**(3): 282-288.

Ramsey, P. S., D. Y. Harris, et al. (2003). "Comparative efficacy and cost of the prostaglandin analogs dinoprostone and misoprostol as labor preinduction agents." Am J Obstet Gynecol **188**(2): 560-565.

Ramsey, P. S., L. Meyer, et al. (2005). "Cardiotocographic abnormalities associated with dinoprostone and misoprostol cervical ripening." Obstet Gynecol **105**(1): 85-90.

Ramsey, P. S., P. L. Ogburn, Jr., et al. (2000). "Effect of vaginal pH on efficacy of misoprostol for cervical ripening and labor induction." Am J Obstet Gynecol **182**(6): 1616-1619.

Ramsey, P. S., K. Savage, et al. (2004). "Vaginal misoprostol versus concentrated oxytocin and vaginal PGE2 for second-trimester labor induction." Obstet Gynecol **104**(1): 138-145.

Reeves, M. F., P. A. Lohr, et al. (2008). "Ultrasonographic endometrial thickness after medical and surgical management of early pregnancy failure." Obstet Gynecol **111**(1): 106-112.

Reynolds, A., D. Ayres-de-Campos, et al. (2005). "How should success be defined when attempting medical resolution of first-trimester missed abortion?" Eur J Obstet Gynecol Reprod Biol **118**(1): 71-76.

Roberts, L. M., C. S. Homer, et al. (2007). "Misoprostol to induce labour: a review of its use in a NSW hospital." Aust N Z J Obstet Gynaecol **47**(4): 291-296.

Robledo, C., J. Zhang, et al. (2007). "Clinical indicators for success of misoprostol treatment after early pregnancy failure." Int J Gynaecol Obstet **99**(1): 46-51.

Rockhead, C., H. Fletcher, et al. (2003). "A comparison of two methods of labor induction with vaginal misoprostol." Int J Gynaecol Obstet **80**(3): 271-277.

Rouzi, A. A. (2003). "Second-trimester pregnancy termination with misoprostol in women with previous cesarean sections." Int J Gynaecol Obstet **80**(3): 317-318.

Rouzi, A. A. (2010). "Abortion failure after illegal use of misoprostol--a case report." Eur J Contracept Reprod Health Care **15**(5): 376-378.

Rowlands, S., R. Bell, et al. (2001). "Misoprostol versus dinoprostone for cervical priming prior to induction of labour in term pregnancy: a randomised controlled trial." Aust N Z J Obstet Gynaecol **41**(2): 145-152.

Ruangchainikhom, W., E. Phongphissanou, et al. (2006). "Effectiveness of 400 or 600 micrograms of vaginal misoprostol for terminations of early pregnancies." J Med Assoc Thai **89**(7): 928-933.

Rust, O. A., M. Greybush, et al. (2001). "Preinduction cervical ripening. A randomized trial of intravaginal misoprostol alone vs. a combination of transcervical Foley balloon and intravaginal misoprostol." J Reprod Med **46**(10): 899-904.

Saha, S., R. Bal, et al. (2006). "Medical abortion in late second trimester--a comparative study with misoprostol through vaginal versus oral followed by vaginal route." J Indian Med Assoc **104**(2): 81-82, 84.

Sahin, H. G., H. A. Sahin, et al. (2001). "Randomized outpatient clinical trial of medical evacuation and surgical curettage in incomplete miscarriage." Eur J Contracept Reprod Health Care **6**(3): 141-144.

Saichua, C. and V. Phupong (2009). "A randomized controlled trial comparing powdery sublingual misoprostol and sublingual misoprostol tablet for management of embryonic death or anembryonic pregnancy." Arch Gynecol Obstet **280**(3): 431-435.

Salakos, N., C. Iavazzo, et al. (2008). "Misoprostol use as a method of medical abortion." Clin Exp Obstet Gynecol **35**(2): 130-132.

Salakos, N., A. Kountouris, et al. (2005). "First-trimester pregnancy termination with 800 microg of vaginal misoprostol every 12 h." Eur J Contracept Reprod Health Care **10**(4): 249-254.

Saleem, S. (2006). "Efficacy of dinoprostone, intracervical foleys and misoprostol in labor induction." J Coll Physicians Surg Pak **16**(4): 276-279.

Sanchez-Ramos, L., C. J. Danner, et al. (2002). "The effect of tablet moistening on labor induction with intravaginal misoprostol: a randomized trial." Obstet Gynecol **99**(6): 1080-1084.

Sanchez-Ramos, L., A. M. Kaunitz, et al. (1993). "Labor induction with the prostaglandin E1 methyl analogue misoprostol versus oxytocin: a randomized trial." Obstet Gynecol **81**(3): 332-336.

Sanchez-Ramos, L., D. E. Peterson, et al. (1998). "Labor induction with prostaglandin E1 misoprostol compared with dinoprostone vaginal insert: a randomized trial." Obstet Gynecol **91**(3): 401-405.

Sanghvi, H., N. Ansari, et al. (2010). "Prevention of postpartum hemorrhage at home birth in Afghanistan." Int J Gynaecol Obstet **108**(3): 276-281.

Saxena, P., S. Salhan, et al. (2003). "Role of sublingual misoprostol for cervical ripening prior to vacuum aspiration in first trimester interruption of pregnancy." Contraception **67**(3): 213-217.

Saxena, P., S. Salhan, et al. (2004). "Comparison between the sublingual and oral route of misoprostol for pre-abortion cervical priming in first trimester abortions." Hum Reprod **19**(1): 77-80.

Saxena, P., S. Salhan, et al. (2006). "Sublingual versus vaginal route of misoprostol for cervical ripening prior to surgical termination of first trimester abortions." Eur J Obstet Gynecol Reprod Biol **125**(1): 109-113.

Saxena, P., N. Sarda, et al. (2008). "A randomised comparison between sublingual, oral and vaginal route of misoprostol for pre-abortion cervical ripening in first-trimester pregnancy termination under local anaesthesia." Aust N Z J Obstet Gynaecol **48**(1): 101-106.

Schaub, B., P. Fuhrer, et al. (1995). "[Randomized study of sulprostone versus misoprostol in the cervical preparation before elective abortion in nulliparous women]." J Gynecol Obstet Biol Reprod (Paris) **24**(5): 505-510.

Schaub, B., P. Fuhrer, et al. (1996). "[Intravaginal misoprostol before induced abortion in nulliparous women]." Contracept Fertil Sex **24**(1): 67-71.

Schuler, L., A. Pastuszak, et al. (1999). "Pregnancy outcome after exposure to misoprostol in Brazil: a prospective, controlled study." Reprod Toxicol **13**(2): 147-151.

Sciscione, A. C., L. Nguyen, et al. (2001). "A randomized comparison of transcervical Foley catheter to intravaginal misoprostol for preinduction cervical ripening." Obstet Gynecol **97**(4): 603-607.

Sciscione, A. C., L. Nguyen, et al. (1998). "Uterine rupture during preinduction cervical ripening with misoprostol in a patient with a previous Caesarean delivery." Aust N Z J Obstet Gynaecol **38**(1): 96-97.

Shah, N., S. I. Azam, et al. (2010). "Sublingual versus vaginal misoprostol in the management of missed miscarriage." J Pak Med Assoc **60**(2): 113-116.

Shakya, R., J. Shrestha, et al. (2010). "Safety and efficacy of misoprostol and dinoprostone as cervical ripening agents." JNMA J Nepal Med Assoc **49**(177): 33-37.

Shankar, M., D. L. Economides, et al. (2007). "Outpatient medical management of missed miscarriage using misoprostol." J Obstet Gynaecol **27**(3): 283-286.

Sharma, D., S. R. Singhal, et al. (2007). "Sublingual misoprostol in management of missed abortion in India." Trop Doct **37**(1): 39-40.

Sharma, S., H. Refaey, et al. (2005). "Oral versus vaginal misoprostol administered one hour before surgical termination of pregnancy: a randomised controlled trial." BJOG **112**(4): 456-460.

Sharma, Y., S. Kumar, et al. (2005). "Evaluation of glyceryl trinitrate, misoprostol, and prostaglandin E2 gel for preinduction cervical ripening in term pregnancy." J Obstet Gynaecol Res **31**(3): 210-215.

Shetty, A., P. Danielian, et al. (2001). "A comparison of oral and vaginal misoprostol tablets in induction of labour at term." BJOG **108**(3): 238-243.

Shetty, A., I. Livingstone, et al. (2003). "Oral misoprostol (100 microg) versus vaginal misoprostol (25 microg) in term labor induction: a randomized comparison." Acta Obstet Gynecol Scand **82**(12): 1103-1106.

Shetty, A., I. Livingstone, et al. (2004). "A randomised comparison of oral misoprostol and vaginal prostaglandin E2 tablets in labour induction at term." BJOG **111**(5): 436-440.

Shetty, A., L. Mackie, et al. (2002). "Sublingual compared with oral misoprostol in term labour induction: a randomised controlled trial." BJOG **109**(6): 645-650.

Shetty, A., K. Stewart, et al. (2002). "Active management of term prelabour rupture of membranes with oral misoprostol." BJOG **109**(12): 1354-1358.

Shojai, R., R. Desbriere, et al. (2004). "[Rectal misoprostol for postpartum hemorrhage]." Gynecol Obstet Fertil **32**(9): 703-707.

Shojai, R., L. Piechon, et al. (2001). "[Rectal administration of misoprostol for delivery induced hemorrhage. Preliminary study]." J Gynecol Obstet Biol Reprod (Paris) **30**(6): 572-575.

Shokry, M., A. Y. Shahin, et al. (2009). "Oral misoprostol reduces vaginal bleeding following surgical evacuation for first trimester spontaneous abortion." Int J Gynaecol Obstet **107**(2): 117-120.

Shwekerela, B., R. Kalumuna, et al. (2007). "Misoprostol for treatment of incomplete abortion at the regional hospital level: results from Tanzania." BJOG **114**(11): 1363-1367.

Sifakis, S., E. Angelakis, et al. (2005). "High-dose misoprostol used in outpatient management of first trimester spontaneous abortion." Arch Gynecol Obstet **272**(3): 183-186.

Silfeler, D. B., B. Tandogan, et al. (2011). "A comparison of misoprostol, controlled-release dinoprostone vaginal insert and oxytocin for cervical ripening." Arch Gynecol Obstet.

Singh, B. M., A. Kriplani, et al. (2005). "Uterocervical laceration during induction of labour with intravaginal misoprostol in a woman with idiopathic thrombocytopenic purpura." J Obstet Gynaecol **25**(1): 75-76.

Singh, G., G. Radhakrishnan, et al. (2009). "Comparison of sublingual misoprostol, intravenous oxytocin, and intravenous methylergometrine in active management of the third stage of labor." Int J Gynaecol Obstet **107**(2): 130-134.

Singh, K., Y. F. Fong, et al. (2003). "A viable alternative to surgical vacuum aspiration: repeated doses of intravaginal misoprostol over 9 hours for medical termination of pregnancies up to eight weeks." BJOG **110**(2): 175-180.

Singh, K., Y. F. Fong, et al. (1998). "Randomized trial to determine optimal dose of vaginal misoprostol for preabortion cervical priming." Obstet Gynecol **92**(5): 795-798.

Singh, K., Y. F. Fong, et al. (1999). "Does an acidic medium enhance the efficacy of vaginal misoprostol for pre-abortion cervical priming?" Hum Reprod **14**(6): 1635-1637.

Singh, K., Y. F. Fong, et al. (1999). "Evacuation interval after vaginal misoprostol for preabortion cervical priming: a randomized trial." Obstet Gynecol **94**(3): 431-434.

Singh, K., Y. F. Fong, et al. (1999). "Vaginal misoprostol for pre-abortion cervical priming: is there an optimal evacuation time interval?" Br J Obstet Gynaecol **106**(3): 266-269.

Sirimai, K., O. Kiriwat, et al. (2002). "Misoprostal use for therapeutic abortion in Siriraj Hospital: the year 2000." J Med Assoc Thai **85**(4): 416-423.

Soltan, M. H., E. El-Gendi, et al. (2007). "Different Doses of Sublingual Misoprostol versus Methylergometrine for the Prevention of Atonic Postpartum Haemorrhage." Int J Health Sci (Qassim) **1**(2): 229-236.

Sparrow, M. J., J. D. Tait, et al. (1998). "Vaginal dinoprostone versus oral misoprostol for predilatation of the cervix in first trimester surgical abortion." Aust N Z J Obstet Gynaecol **38**(1): 64-68.

Srikhao, N. and Y. Tannirandorn (2005). "A comparison of vaginal misoprostol 800 microg versus 400 microg for anembryonic pregnancy: a randomized comparative trial." J Med Assoc Thai **88 Suppl 2**: S41-47.

Srisomboon, J., W. Piyamongkol, et al. (1997). "Comparison of intracervical and intravaginal misoprostol for cervical ripening and labour induction in patients with an unfavourable cervix." J Med Assoc Thai **80**(3): 189-194.

Srisomboon, J. and S. Pongpisuttinun (1998). "Efficacy of intracervicovaginal misoprostol in second-trimester pregnancy termination: a comparison between live and dead fetuses." J Obstet Gynaecol Res **24**(1): 1-5.

Srisomboon, J., T. Tongsong, et al. (1997). "Termination of second-trimester pregnancy with intracervicovaginal misoprostol." J Med Assoc Thai **80**(4): 242-246.

Srisomboon, J., T. Tongsong, et al. (1996). "Preinduction cervical ripening with intravaginal prostaglandin E1 methyl analogue misoprostol: a randomized controlled trial." J Obstet Gynaecol Res **22**(2): 119-124.

Stitely, M. L., J. Browning, et al. (2000). "Outpatient cervical ripening with intravaginal misoprostol." Obstet Gynecol **96**(5 Pt 1): 684-688.

Su, L. L., A. Biswas, et al. (2005). "A prospective, randomized comparison of vaginal misoprostol versus intra-amniotic prostaglandins for midtrimester termination of pregnancy." Am J Obstet Gynecol **193**(4): 1410-1414.

Sundaram, S., J. P. Diaz, et al. (2009). "Rectal misoprostol vs 15-methyl prostaglandin F2alpha for retained placenta after second-trimester delivery." Am J Obstet Gynecol **200**(5): e24-26.

Surbek, D. V., P. M. Fehr, et al. (1999). "Oral misoprostol for third stage of labor: a randomized placebo-controlled trial." Obstet Gynecol **94**(2): 255-258.

Szczesny, W., M. Kjollesdal, et al. (2006). "Bishop score and the outcome of labor induction with misoprostol." Acta Obstet Gynecol Scand **85**(5): 579-582.

Szczesny, W. and L. Sandvik (2009). "Pre-induction cervical ripening with 25 microg and 50 microg vaginal misoprostol in 181 nulliparous parturients." J Matern Fetal Neonatal Med **22**(3): 265-268.

Tabowei, T. O. and V. O. Oboro (2003). "Low dose intravaginal misoprostol versus intracervical baloon catheter for pre-induction cervical ripening." East Afr Med J **80**(2): 91-94.

Tam, W. H., M. H. Tsui, et al. (2005). "Long-term reproductive outcome subsequent to medical versus surgical treatment for miscarriage." Hum Reprod **20**(12): 3355-3359.

Tan, T. C., S. Y. Yan, et al. (2010). "A randomised controlled trial of low-dose misoprostol and dinoprostone vaginal pessaries for cervical priming." BJOG **117**(10): 1270-1277.

Taner, C. E., U. Nayki, et al. (2004). "Misoprostol for medical management of first-trimester pregnancy failure." Int J Gynaecol Obstet **86**(3): 407-408.

Tang, O. S. and P. C. Ho (2001). "Pilot study on the use of sublingual misoprostol for medical abortion." Contraception **64**(5): 315-317.

Tang, O. S., W. N. Lau, et al. (2004). "A prospective randomised comparison of sublingual and vaginal misoprostol in second trimester termination of pregnancy." BJOG **111**(9): 1001-1005.

Tang, O. S., W. N. Lau, et al. (2003). "A prospective randomized study to compare the use of repeated doses of vaginal with sublingual misoprostol in the management of first trimester silent miscarriages." Hum Reprod **18**(1): 176-181.

Tang, O. S., B. Y. Miao, et al. (2002). "Pilot study on the use of repeated doses of sublingual misoprostol in termination of pregnancy up to 12 weeks gestation: efficacy and acceptability." Hum Reprod **17**(3): 654-658.

Tang, O. S., K. H. Mok, et al. (2004). "A randomized study comparing the use of sublingual to vaginal misoprostol for pre-operative cervical priming prior to surgical termination of pregnancy in the first trimester." Hum Reprod **19**(5): 1101-1104.

Tang, O. S., C. Y. Ong, et al. (2006). "A randomized trial to compare the use of sublingual misoprostol with or without an additional 1 week course for the management of first trimester silent miscarriage." Hum Reprod **21**(1): 189-192.

Tang, O. S., K. S. Wong, et al. (1999). "Pilot study on the use of repeated doses of misoprostol in termination of pregnancy at less than 9 weeks of gestation." Adv Contracept **15**(3): 211-216.

Tanha, F. D., M. Feizi, et al. (2010). "Sublingual versus vaginal misoprostol for the management of missed abortion." J Obstet Gynaecol Res **36**(3): 525-532.

Tanir, H. M., T. Sener, et al. (2008). "Digital and transvaginal ultrasound cervical assessment for prediction of successful labor induction." Int J Gynaecol Obstet **100**(1): 52-55.

Tarim, E., E. Kilicdag, et al. (2005). "Second-trimester pregnancy termination with oral misoprostol in women who have had one cesarean section." Int J Gynaecol Obstet **90**(1): 84-85.

Taylor, J., A. Diop, et al. (2011). "Oral misoprostol as an alternative to surgical management for incomplete abortion in Ghana." Int J Gynaecol Obstet **112**(1): 40-44.

Thornburg, L. L., D. Grace, et al. (2010). "Placement of laminaria tents does not improve time to delivery in patients undergoing second trimester labor induction with misoprostol." J Matern Fetal Neonatal Med **23**(8): 928-931.

Todd, C. S., M. Soler, et al. (2002). "Buccal misoprostol as cervical preparation for second trimester pregnancy termination." Contraception **65**(6): 415-418.

Toppozada, M. K., M. Y. Anwar, et al. (1997). "Oral or vaginal misoprostol for induction of labor." Int J Gynaecol Obstet **56**(2): 135-139.

Tukur, J., N. I. Umar, et al. (2007). "Comparison of emergency caesarean section to misoprostol induction for the delivery of antepartum eclamptic patients: a pilot study." Niger J Med **16**(4): 364-367.

Turan, C., N. Koc, et al. (2003). "Misoprostol administration in first-trimester pregnancies with embryonic demise reduces uterine arterial blood flow." J Matern Fetal Neonatal Med **14**(4): 226-228.

Uludag, S., F. Salihoglu Saricali, et al. (2005). "A comparison of oral and vaginal misoprostol for induction of labor." Eur J Obstet Gynecol Reprod Biol **122**(1): 57-60.

Umar, N. I., M. A. Abdul, et al. (2008). "Disseminated intravascular coagulation following induction of labour with misoprostol: a case report." Niger J Med **17**(2): 156-158.

Urban, R., A. Lemancewicz, et al. (2003). "Misoprostol and dinoprostone therapy for labor induction: a Doppler comparison of uterine and fetal hemodynamic effects." Eur J Obstet Gynecol Reprod Biol **106**(1): 20-24.

Vaid, A., V. Dadhwal, et al. (2009). "A randomized controlled trial of prophylactic sublingual misoprostol versus intramuscular methyl-ergometrine versus intramuscular 15-methyl PGF2alpha in active management of third stage of labor." Arch Gynecol Obstet **280**(6): 893-897.

van Bogaert, L. J. (2008). "Termination of pregnancy with misoprostol in the scarred uterus." Int J Gynaecol Obstet **100**(1): 80-81.

van Bogaert, L. J. and A. Misra (2010). "Anthropometric characteristics and success rates of oral or vaginal misoprostol for pregnancy termination in the first and second trimesters." Int J Gynaecol Obstet **109**(3): 213-215.

van Bogaert, L. J. and T. M. Sedibe (2007). "Efficacy of a single misoprostol regimen in the first and second trimester termination of pregnancy." J Obstet Gynaecol **27**(5): 510-512.

Van Mensel, K., F. Claerhout, et al. (2009). "A randomized controlled trial of misoprostol and sulprostone to end pregnancy after fetal death." Obstet Gynecol Int **2009**: 496320.

Vejborg, T. S., L. Nilas, et al. (2007). "Medical management of first trimester miscarriage according to ultrasonographic findings." Acta Obstet Gynecol Scand **86**(5): 604-609.

Vejborg, T. S., C. Rorbye, et al. (2006). "Management of first trimester spontaneous abortion with 800 or 400 microg vaginal misoprostol." Int J Gynaecol Obstet **92**(3): 268-269.

Velazco, A., L. Varela, et al. (2000). "Misoprostol for abortion up to 9 weeks' gestation in adolescents." Eur J Contracept Reprod Health Care **5**(4): 227-233.

Vengalil, S. R., D. A. Guinn, et al. (1998). "A randomized trial of misoprostol and extra-amniotic saline infusion for cervical ripening and labor induction." Obstet Gynecol **91**(5 Pt 1): 774-779.

Vimala, N., V. Dadhwal, et al. (2004). "Sublingual misoprostol for second-trimester abortion." Int J Gynaecol Obstet **84**(1): 89-90.

Vimala, N., S. Mittal, et al. (2005). "Cervical priming with sublingual misoprostol vs. 15-methyl-prostaglandin F2alpha prior to surgical abortion." Int J Gynaecol Obstet **88**(2): 134-137.

Vimala, N., S. Mittal, et al. (2003). "Sublingual misoprostol for preabortion cervical ripening in first-trimester pregnancy termination." Contraception **67**(4): 295-297.

Vimala, N., S. Mittal, et al. (2004). "Sublingual misoprostol before first trimester abortion: a comparative study using two dose regimens." Indian J Med Sci **58**(2): 54-61.

Vimala, N., S. Mittal, et al. (2006). "Sublingual misoprostol versus oxytocin infusion to reduce blood loss at cesarean section." Int J Gynaecol Obstet **92**(2): 106-110.

Vimala, N., S. Mittal, et al. (2004). "Sublingual misoprostol versus methylergometrine for active management of the third stage of labor." Int J Gynaecol Obstet **87**(1): 1-5.

von Hertzen, H., G. Piaggio, et al. (2007). "Efficacy of two intervals and two routes of administration of misoprostol for termination of early pregnancy: a randomised controlled equivalence trial." Lancet **369**(9577): 1938-1946.

von Hertzen, H., G. Piaggio, et al. (2009). "Comparison of vaginal and sublingual misoprostol for second trimester abortion: randomized controlled equivalence trial." Hum Reprod **24**(1): 106-112.

Wakabayashi, M., M. Tretiak, et al. (1998). "Intravaginal misoprostol for medical evacuation of first trimester missed abortion." Prim Care Update Ob Gyns **5**(4): 176.

Walley, R. L., J. B. Wilson, et al. (2000). "A double-blind placebo controlled randomised trial of misoprostol and oxytocin in the management of the third stage of labour." BJOG **107**(9): 1111-1115.

Walraven, G., J. Blum, et al. (2005). "Misoprostol in the management of the third stage of labour in the home delivery setting in rural Gambia: a randomised controlled trial." BJOG **112**(9): 1277-1283.

Walraven, G., Y. Dampha, et al. (2004). "Misoprostol in the treatment of postpartum haemorrhage in addition to routine management: a placebo randomised controlled trial." BJOG **111**(9): 1014-1017.

Wang, Z., W. Li, et al. (1998). "Cervical ripening in the third trimester of pregnancy with intravaginal misoprostol: a double-blind, randomized, placebo-controlled study." J Tongji Med Univ **18**(3): 183-186.

Weeks, A., G. Alia, et al. (2005). "A randomized trial of misoprostol compared with manual vacuum aspiration for incomplete abortion." Obstet Gynecol **106**(3): 540-547.

Whitecar, P. W., A. Zweifel, et al. (1999). "Failed second-trimester misoprostol termination responding to vaginal instillation of citric acid." Obstet Gynecol **94**(5 Pt 2): 839.

Widmer, M., J. Blum, et al. (2010). "Misoprostol as an adjunct to standard uterotonics for treatment of post-partum haemorrhage: a multicentre, double-blind randomised trial." Lancet **375**(9728): 1808-1813.

Wiebe, E. R. and M. J. Rawling (1998). "Vaginal misoprostol before first trimester abortion." Int J Gynaecol Obstet **60**(2): 175-176.

Wing, D. A. (2008). "Misoprostol vaginal insert compared with dinoprostone vaginal insert: a randomized controlled trial." Obstet Gynecol **112**(4): 801-812.

Wing, D. A., M. J. Fassett, et al. (2004). "A comparison of orally administered misoprostol to intravenous oxytocin for labor induction in women with favorable cervical examinations." Am J Obstet Gynecol **190**(6): 1689-1694; discussion 1694-1686.

Wing, D. A., D. Ham, et al. (1999). "A comparison of orally administered misoprostol with vaginally administered misoprostol for cervical ripening and labor induction." Am J Obstet Gynecol **180**(5): 1155-1160.

Wing, D. A., M. M. Jones, et al. (1995). "A comparison of misoprostol and prostaglandin E2 gel for preinduction cervical ripening and labor induction." Am J Obstet Gynecol **172**(6): 1804-1810.

Wing, D. A., G. Ortiz-Omphroy, et al. (1997). "A comparison of intermittent vaginal administration of misoprostol with continuous dinoprostone for cervical ripening and labor induction." Am J Obstet Gynecol **177**(3): 612-618.

Wing, D. A., M. R. Park, et al. (2000). "A randomized comparison of oral and intravaginal misoprostol for labor induction." Obstet Gynecol **95**(6 Pt 1): 905-908.

Wing, D. A. and R. H. Paul (1996). "A comparison of differing dosing regimens of vaginally administered misoprostol for preinduction cervical ripening and labor induction." Am J Obstet Gynecol **175**(1): 158-164.

Wing, D. A. and R. H. Paul (1998). "Induction of labor with misoprostol for premature rupture of membranes beyond thirty-six weeks' gestation." Am J Obstet Gynecol 179(1): 94-99.

Wing, D. A., B. L. Powers, et al. (2008). "Determining dose and endpoints of a controlled-release misoprostol vaginal insert for a phase III trial." J Reprod Med 53(9): 695-696.

Wing, D. A., S. Tran, et al. (2002). "Factors affecting the likelihood of successful induction after intravaginal misoprostol application for cervical ripening and labor induction." Am J Obstet Gynecol 186(6): 1237-1240; discussion 1240-1233.

Winikoff, B., R. Dabash, et al. (2010). "Treatment of post-partum haemorrhage with sublingual misoprostol versus oxytocin in women not exposed to oxytocin during labour: a double-blind, randomised, non-inferiority trial." Lancet 375(9710): 210-216.

Wolf, S. B., L. Sanchez-Ramos, et al. (2005). "Sublingual misoprostol for labor induction: a randomized clinical trial." Obstet Gynecol 105(2): 365-371.

Wong, K. S., C. S. Ngai, et al. (1996). "Termination of second trimester pregnancy with gemeprost and misoprostol: a randomized double-blind placebo-controlled trial." Contraception 54(1): 23-25.

Wong, K. S., C. S. Ngai, et al. (1998). "Vaginal misoprostol compared with vaginal gemeprost in termination of second trimester pregnancy. A randomized trial." Contraception 58(4): 207-210.

Wong, K. S., C. S. Ngai, et al. (2000). "A comparison of two regimens of intravaginal misoprostol for termination of second trimester pregnancy: a randomized comparative trial." Hum Reprod 15(3): 709-712.

Wood, S. L. and P. H. Brain (2002). "Medical management of missed abortion: a randomized clinical trial." Obstet Gynecol 99(4): 563-566.

Wright-Francis, D. L., B. D. Raynor, et al. (1998). "Misoprostol in second trimester termination of pregnancy." Prim Care Update Ob Gyns 5(4): 176.

Yacoub, A. and M. J. Martel (2002). "Pregnancy with primary dilated cardiomyopathy." Obstet Gynecol 99(5 Pt 2): 928-930.

Yapar, E. G., S. Senoz, et al. (1996). "Second trimester pregnancy termination including fetal death: comparison of five different methods." Eur J Obstet Gynecol Reprod Biol **69**(2): 97-102.

Yilmaz, B., I. E. Ertas, et al. (2010). "Moistening of misoprostol tablets with acetic acid prior to vaginal administration for mid-trimester termination of anomalous pregnancy: A randomised comparison of three regimens." Eur J Contracept Reprod Health Care **15**(1): 54-59.

Yilmaz, B., S. Kelekci, et al. (2005). "Misoprostol moistened with acetic acid or saline for second trimester pregnancy termination: a randomized prospective double-blind trial." Hum Reprod **20**(11): 3067-3071.

Yilmaz, B., S. Kelekci, et al. (2007). "Randomized comparison of second trimester pregnancy termination utilizing saline moistened or dry misoprostol." Arch Gynecol Obstet **276**(5): 511-516.

Zachariah, E. S., M. Naidu, et al. (2006). "Oral misoprostol in the third stage of labor." Int J Gynaecol Obstet **92**(1): 23-26.

Zahran, K. M., A. Y. Shahin, et al. (2009). "Sublingual versus vaginal misoprostol for induction of labor at term: a randomized prospective placebo-controlled study." J Obstet Gynaecol Res **35**(6): 1054-1060.

Zalanyi, S. (1998). "Vaginal misoprostol alone is effective in the treatment of missed abortion." Br J Obstet Gynaecol **105**(9): 1026-1028.

Zeqiri, F., M. Pacarada, et al. (2010). "Missed abortion and application of misoprostol." Med Arh **64**(3): 151-153.

Zeteroglu, S., Y. Engin-Ustun, et al. (2006). "A prospective randomized study comparing misoprostol and oxytocin for premature rupture of membranes at term." J Matern Fetal Neonatal Med **19**(5): 283-287.

Zeteroglu, S., G. H. Sahin, et al. (2006). "Induction of labor with misoprostol in pregnancies with advanced maternal age." Eur J Obstet Gynecol Reprod Biol **129**(2): 140-144.

Zeteroglu, S., H. G. Sahin, et al. (2006). "Induction of labor in great grandmultipara with misoprostol." Eur J Obstet Gynecol Reprod Biol **126**(1): 27-32.

Zhang, J., J. M. Gilles, et al. (2005). "A comparison of medical management with misoprostol and surgical management for early pregnancy failure." N Engl J Med **353**(8): 761-769.

Zikopoulos, K. A., E. G. Papanikolaou, et al. (2002). "Early pregnancy termination with vaginal misoprostol before and after 42 days gestation." Hum Reprod **17**(12): 3079-3083.

Zuberi, N. F., J. Durocher, et al. (2008). "Misoprostol in addition to routine treatment of postpartum hemorrhage: a hospital-based randomized-controlled trial in Karachi, Pakistan." BMC Pregnancy Childbirth **8**: 40.

6.2 References

1. http://de.wikipedia.org/wiki/Misoprostol
2. http://www.misoprostol.org/File/offlabeluse.php
3. http://www.kompendium.ch
4. http://www.sappinfo.ch
5. Tang, O. S. and P. C. Ho (2006). "The pharmacokinetics and different regimens of misoprostol in early first-trimester medical abortion." Contraception **74**(1): 26-30.
6. BJOG 2005: BJOG: an International Journal of Obstetrics and Gynaecology
March 2005, Vol. 112, pp. 269-272
7. Tang, O. S., H. Schweer, et al. (2002). "Pharmacokinetics of different routes of administration of misoprostol." Hum Reprod **17**(2): 332-336.
8. Lengyel, Pildner von Steinberg 2001: Lengyel E., Pildner von Steinberg, S. (2001). "Die Physiologie der Zervixreifung". Gynäkologie **34**: 708-714.
9. Breckwoldt et al. 2007: Breckwoldt, M.; Kaufmann, M.; Pfleiderer, A., Gynäkologie und Geburtshilfe (2007), 5. Auflage, Georg Thieme Verlag, Stuttgart/New York, p. 425
10. Kapp, N., P. A. Lohr, et al. (2010). "Cervical preparation for first trimester surgical abortion." Cochrane Database Syst Rev(2): CD007207.
11. http://www.who.int/medicines/publications/essentialmedicines/Updated_sixteenth_adult_list_en.pdf
12. Ng, P. S., C. Y. Lai, et al. (2007). "A double-blind randomized controlled trial of oral misoprostol and intramuscular syntometrine in the management of the third stage of labor." Gynecol Obstet Invest **63**(1): 55-60.
13. Karkanis, S. G., D. Caloia, et al. (2002). "Randomized controlled trial of rectal misoprostol versus oxytocin in third stage management." J Obstet Gynaecol Can **24**(2): 149-154.

14. Hofmeyr, G. J., V. C. Nikodem, et al. (1998). "A randomised placebo controlled trial of oral misoprostol in the third stage of labour." Br J Obstet Gynaecol **105**(9): 971-975.
15. Mousa, H. A. and Z. Alfirevic (2007). "Treatment for primary postpartum haemorrhage." Cochrane Database Syst Rev(1): CD003249.
16. Langer, B., E. Boudier, et al. (2004). "[Obstetrical management in the event of persistent or worsening postpartum hemorrhage despite initial measures]." J Gynecol Obstet Biol Reprod (Paris) **33**(8 Suppl): 4S73-74S79.
17. http://www.misoprostol.org
18. Goldberg, A. B., M. B. Greenberg, et al. (2001). "Misoprostol and pregnancy." N Engl J Med **344**(1): 38-47.
19. http://www.novartis.ch/research/drug-discovery.shtml
20. Ausführung der Schweizerischen Kantonsapothekenvereinigung und der Swissmedic 2006: Ausführung der Schweizerischen Kantonsapothekenvereinigung und der Swissmedic betreffend des Einsatzes von Arzneimitteln im Sinne des off-label use; Basel 24. 7. 2006)
21. Expertenbrief No. 23, 2007: Expertenbrief No. 23: „Off-label use" von Arzneimitteln in Gynäkologie und Geburtshilfe; D. Surbek, S. Heinzl, W. Holzgreve, J. Seydoux, W. Pletscher), 2007
22. http://www.cochrane-handbook.org/
23. Dodd, J. M. and C. A. Crowther (2010). "Misoprostol for induction of labour to terminate pregnancy in the second or third trimester for women with a foetal anomaly or after intrauterine foetal death." Cochrane Database Syst Rev(4): CD004901.
24. Khan, R. U., H. El-Refaey, et al. (2004). "Oral, rectal, and vaginal pharmacokinetics of misoprostol." Obstet Gynecol **103**(5 Pt 1): 866-870.
25. Alfirevic, Z. and A. Weeks (2006). "Oral misoprostol for induction of labour." Cochrane Database Syst Rev(2): CD001338.

26. Neilson, J. P., G. M. Gyte, et al. (2010). "Medical treatments for incomplete miscarriage (less than 24 weeks)." <u>Cochrane Database Syst Rev</u>(1): CD007223.
27. Hofmeyr, G. J., A. M. Gulmezoglu, et al. (2010). "Vaginal misoprostol for cervical ripening and induction of labour." <u>Cochrane Database Syst Rev</u>(10): CD000941.

7. Abbreviations

ADR	Adverse drug reaction
AUC curve	Area under the plasma-concentration-versus-time
CI	Confidence interval
CS	Caesarean section
FDA	Food and Drug Administration
FHRch	Foetal heart-rate changes
F/SH	Fever and/or shivering
GIT	Gastrointestinal ADR
HMG	Heilmittelgesetz
HS	Hyperstimulation syndrome
IUPAC	International Union of Pure and Applied Chemistry
NICU	Neonatal intensive care unit
NO	Nitric oxide
NSAID	Non-steroidal antirheumatics
PGE	Prostaglandin E
PGF	Prostaglandin F
PGE-R	Prostaglandin E receptor
PID	Pelvic inflammatory disease
PGF-R	Prostaglandin F receptor
PMID	PubMed Unique Identifier

PPH		Postpartum haemorrhage

RCT		Randomised controlled trial

8. Appendix

Included RCT

	Cervical ripening and labour induction	Abortion induction	Prevention of PPH
RCT total	**218**	**116**	**64**
Misoprostol vs. placebo or no treatment			
Buccal misoprostol vs. placebo	0	0	1
Oral misoprostol vs. no/standard treatment	2	1	3
Oral misoprostol vs. placebo	7	0	6
Sublingual misoprostol vs. no/standard treatment	1	3	2
Sublingual misoprostol vs. placebo	2	0	3
Vaginal misoprostol vs. no/standard treatment	2	2	0
Vaginal misoprostol vs. placebo	10	4	0
Vaginal-oral misoprostol vs. placebo	1	0	0
Misoprostol (oral, rectal, sublingual) vs. placebo	0	0	2
Misoprostol: different applications			
Buccal misoprostol vs. vaginal misoprostol	1	0	0
Oral misoprostol vs. sublingual misoprostol	3	3	0
Oral misoprostol vs. vaginal misoprostol	27	10	1
Oral misoprostol vs. rectal misoprostol	0	0	1
Vaginal misoprostol vs. oral-vaginal misoprostol	0	2	0
Vaginal misoprostol vs. oral misoprostol vs. vaginal-oral misoprostol	1	1	0
Vaginal misoprostol vs. buccal-vaginal misoprostol	0	1	0
Sublingual misoprostol vs. oral misoprostol vs. vaginal misoprostol	1	3	0
Vaginal misoprostol vs. cervical misoprostol	2	0	0
Vaginal misoprostol vs. rectal misoprostol	0	1	1
Misoprostol: different doses / regimens			
Oral misoprostol (25 vs. 50 µg)	1	0	0
Oral misoprostol (50 vs. 100 µg)	1	0	0
Oral misoprostol (200 vs. 400 µg)	1	0	0
Oral misoprostol (400 µg normal vs. 400 µg slow release vs. 800 µg slow release)	1	0	0
Oral misoprostol (600 vs. 1200 µg)	0	2	0
Oral misoprostol (every 3 h vs. every 6 h)	1	2	0
Oral misoprostol (every 4 h vs. every 6 h)	1	0	0
Oral misoprostol (17 vs. 10 h before abortion)	1	0	0
Sublingual misoprostol (50 vs. 100 µg)	1	0	0

Sublingual misoprostol (100 vs.200 µg)	0	1	0
Sublingual misoprostol (every 3 h vs. every 3 and 24 h)	0	1	0
Sublingual misoprostol (powder) v. sublingual misoprostol (tablet)	0	1	0
Vaginal misoprostol (25 vs.50 µg)	7	0	0
Vaginal misoprostol (50 vs.100 µg)	2	0	0
Vaginal misoprostol (every 3 h) vs. vaginal misoprostol (every 6 h)	1	0	0
Vaginal misoprostol (200 vs. 400 vs.600 vs. 800 µg)	1	0	0
Vaginal misoprostol (200 vs. 400 µg)	1	2	0
Vaginal misoprostol (200 vs.400 vs. 800 µg)	0	1	0
Vaginal misoprostol (400 vs. 600 µg)	1	3	0
Vaginal misoprostol (400 vs. 800 µg)	0	1	0
Vaginal misoprostol (400 vs.600 vs. 800 µg)	1	3	0
Vaginal misoprostol (600 vs. 800 µg)	0	1	0
Vaginal misoprostol (600 vs. 1000 µg)	0	1	0
Vaginal misoprostol (every 6 h) vs. vaginal misoprostol (every 12 h)	0	3	0
Vaginal misoprostol (moistened with water) vs. vaginal misoprostol (moistened with acetic acid)	1	1	0
Vaginal misoprostol (dry) vs. vaginal misoprostol (moistened with acetic acid)	2	0	0
Vaginal misoprostol (dry) vs. vaginal misoprostol (moistened with water)	0	4	0
Vaginal misoprostol (outpatient administration) vs. vaginal misoprostol (inpatient administration)	1	1	0
Vaginal misoprostol (tablet) vs. vaginal misoprostol (gel)	1	1	0
Vaginal misoprostol (vaginal tablet) vs. vaginal misoprostol (oral tablet)	1	0	0
Misoprostol vs. other uterotonics			
Buccal misoprostol plus oxytocin vs. oxytocin alone	0	0	1
Cervical misoprostol vs. PGE2	1	1	0
Cervical misoprostol vs. PGF2alpha	0	1	0
Oral misoprostol vs. ergometrine	0	0	1
Oral misoprostol vs. methylergometrine	0	0	3
Oral misoprostol alone vs. IMN alone vs. IMN plus oral misoprostol	1	0	0
Oral misoprostol alone vs. oral misoprostol plus Foley catheter vs. PGE2	1	0	0

Oral misoprostol alone vs. oral misoprostol plus oxytocin	1	0	0
Oral misoprostol alone vs. oral misoprostol plus oxytocin vs. oxytocin alone vs. oxytocin plus methylergonovine maleate	0	0	1
Oral misoprostol vs. gemeprost	1	0	0
Oral misoprostol plus gemeprost vs. gemeprost alone	0	1	0
Oral misoprostol vs. oxytocin	6	0	10
Oral misoprostol vs. oxytocin vs. ergometrine	0	0	1
Oral misoprostol plus oxytocin vs. oxytocin alone	0	0	1
Oral misoprostol vs. Foley catheter plus oxytocin	1	0	0
Oral misoprostol vs. PGE 2	8	0	0
Oral misoprostol vs. PGE2 vs. Foley catheter	1	0	0
Oral misoprostol vs. sulprostone	1	0	0
Oral misoprostol vs. syntometrin	0	0	3
Oral misoprostol vs. vaginal misoprostol vs. PGE2	1	0	0
Oral misoprostol vs. vaginal misoprostol vs. PGE2 vs. PGF2alpha	1	0	0
Oral misoprostol vs. vaginal-oral misoprostol vs. PGE2	1	0	0
Oral misoprostol vs. vaginal misoprostol vs. PGF2alpha plus oxytocin	0	1	0
Oral misoprostol vs. PGF2alpha	0	1	0
Oxytocin plus vaginal misoprostol vs. oxytocin alone	2	0	0
Rectal misoprostol vs. methylergometrine	0	0	1
Rectal misoprostol vs. oxytocin	0	0	5
Rectal misoprostol alone vs. rectal misoprostol plus oxytocin vs. oxytocin alone vs. oxytocin plus methylergometrine	0	0	1
Rectal misoprostol vs. PGF2alpha	0	0	1
Rectal misoprostol vs. placebo	0	0	1
Rectal misoprostol vs. syntometine	0	0	2
Rectal misoprostol vs. syntometrine plus syntocinon	0	0	1
Sublingual misoprostol vs. 15-M-PGF2alpha (Prostodin)	1	0	0
Sublingual misoprostol methylergometrin	0	0	2
Sublingual misoprostol vs. methylergometrin vs. 15-methyl PGF2alpha	0	0	1
Sublingual misoprostol plus oxytocin vs. oxytocin alone	0	0	1
Sublingual misoprostol vs. oxytocin	0	0	4

Sublingual misoprostol vs. oxytocin vs. methylergometrin	0	0	1
Sublingual misoprostol vs. syntometrine	0	0	1
Vaginal misoprostol alone vs. IMN plus vaginal misoprostol vs. IMN	1	0	0
Vaginal misoprostol plus IMN vs. vaginal misoprostol plus placebo	1	0	0
Vaginal misoprostol plus placebo vs. sodium nitroprusside plus placebo	1	0	0
Vaginal misoprostol vs. Foley catheter plus oxytocin	2	0	0
Vaginal misoprostol vs. Foley catheter plus PGE2	1	0	0
Vaginal misoprostol vs. Foley catheter vs. Foley catheter plus PGE2	1	0	0
Vaginal misoprostol alone vs. Foley catheter plus vaginal misoprostol vs. Foley catheter plus PGE2	1	0	0
Vaginal misoprostol vs. gemeprost	3	4	0
Vaginal misoprostol vs. IMN	6	0	0
Vaginal misoprostol vs. IMN vs. Dilapan-S	1	0	0
Vaginal misoprostol plus placebo vs. vaginal misoprostol plus IMN	0	1	0
Vaginal misoprostol vs. isosorbite dinitrate	1	0	0
Vaginal misoprostol alone vs. vaginal misoprostol plus isosorbite dinitrate	0	1	0
Vaginal misoprostol vs. oxytocin	12	0	0
Vaginal misoprostol plus oxytocin vs. misoprostol alone	0	1	0
Vaginal misoprostol (high vs. low dose) plus oxytocin	0	1	0
Vaginal misoprostol vs. oxytocin vs. Foley catheter	1	0	0
Vaginal misoprostol vs. PGE2	35	2	0
Vaginal misoprostol vs. PGE2 plus oxytocin	1	2	0
Vaginal misoprostol vs. PGE2 vs. glyceryl trinitrate	1	1	0
Vaginal misoprostol vs. PGF2alpha	0	2	0
Vaginal misoprostol vs. intrauterine instillation of hypertonic saline plus PGF analogue	0	1	0
Vaginal misoprostol vs. extraamniotic ethacridine lactate vs. PGE2 vs. oxytocin vs. baloon insertion	0	1	0
Vaginal misoprostol vs. sulprostone	0	1	0
Vaginal-oral misoprostol vs. PGE2 plus oxytocin	1	0	0
Misoprostol vs. mechanical methods			
Oral misoprostol vs. surgical evacuation	1	0	0
Laminaria plus (oral misoprostol vs. vaginal misoprostol vs. placebo)	0	7	0

Laminaria plus (buccal misoprostol vs. placebo)	1	0	0
Sublingual misoprostol vs. surgical evacuation	1	0	0
Vaginal misoprostol vs. Foley catheter	0	1	1
Vaginal misoprostol vs. Foley catheter plus oral misoprostol	7	0	0
Vaginal misoprostol vs. Foley catheter plus vaginal misoprostol	1	0	0
Vaginal misoprostol vs. Foley catheter vs. Foley catheter plus vaginal misoprostol	1	0	0
Vaginal misoprostol vs. Foley catheter with extra-amniotic saline solution infusion	2	0	0
Vaginal misoprostol vs. laminaria	3	0	0
Vaginal misoprostol alone vs. vaginal misoprostol plus laminaria	2	0	0
Vaginal misoprostol vs. surgical evacuation	0	3	0
Vaginal misoprostol plus surgical evacuation vs. surgical evacuation plus placebo	0	10	1
Vaginal misoprostol vs. emergency CS	1	0	0
Vaginal-oral misoprostol alone vs. vaginal-oral misoprostol plus Foley catheter with extraamniotic ethacridine lactate plus / minus oxytocin	1	0	0
Other			
Oral misoprostol alone vs. oral misoprostol plus diclofenac	0	1	0
Oral misoprostol plus placebo vs. ZB 11 plus placebo (traditional tibetan medicine)	1	0	0
Vaginal misoprostol vs. electroacupuncture	0	0	1
Vaginal misoprostol plus loperamide and acetaminophen vs. vaginal misoprostol alone	1	0	0
Vaginal misoprostol plus placebo vs. vaginal misoprostol plus letrozole	0	1	0

Maternal ADR with misoprostol prior to surgical termination

	Cervical ripening and labour induction		
ADR	N women	ADR (%)	CI 95%
No ADR	364	290 (79.7)	75.2 - 83.5
Gastrointestinal ADR	9'435	1'847 (19.6)	18.8 - 20.4
Fever and/or shivering	7'051	720 (10.2)	9.5 - 10.9
Infection*	6'524	16 (0.2)	0.2 - 0.4
Maternal death	21'474	0 (0.0)	0.0 - 0.0
Other ADR	4'376	212 (4.8)	4.2 - 5.5

*(endometritis, chorioamnionitis, PID)

Maternal ADR: Sublingual application

	Cervical ripening and labour induction			Abortion induction			Prevention of PPH			All indications		
ADR	N women	ADR (%)	CI 95%	N women	ADR (%)	CI 95%	N women	ADR (%)	CI 95%	N women	ADR (%)	CI 95%
Gastro-intestinal ADR	1'642	550 (33.5)	31.3 - 35.8	5'235	3'142 (60.0)	58.7 - 61.3	3'111	447 (14.4)	13.2 - 15.6	9'988	4'139 (41.4)	40.5 - 42.4
Fever and/or shivering	1'672	213 (12.7)	11.2 - 14.4	5'156	2'474 (48.0)	46.6 - 49.3	4'509	3'043 (67.5)	66.1 - 68.8	11'337	5'730 (50.5)	49.6 -51.5
Infection*	1'203	18 (1.5)	0.9 - 2.4	n. e.			n. e.			1'203	18 (1.5)	0.9 - 2.4
Maternal death	3'303	0 (0.0)	0.0 - 0.1	5'386	0 (0.0)	0.0 - 0.1	4'667	4 (0.1)	0.0 - 0.2	13'356	4 (0.0)	0.0 - 0.1
Other ADR	833	78 (9.4)	7.6 - 11.5	1'059	389 (36.7)	33.9 - 39.7	2'382	155 (6.5)	5.6 - 7.6	4'274	622 (14.6)	13.5 - 15.6

*(endometritis, chorioamnionitis, PID)

Maternal ADR: Rectal application

	Prevention of PPH		
ADR	N women	ADR (%)	CI 95%
Gastrointestinal ADR	1'850	187 (10.1)	3.0 - 9.6
Fever and/or shivering	1'842	729 (39.6)	4.0 - 7.3
Infection	n. e.		
Maternal death	3'268	0(0.0)	0.0 – 0.0
Other ADR	206	160 (77.7)	40.9 - 56.2

* (endometritis, chorioamnionitis, PID)

In cervical ripening, labour and abortion induction there were not enough cases with rectal application to be evaluated.

Birth outcome with misoprostol prior to surgical termination

	Cervical ripening and/or labour induction		
Event	N women	Event (%)	CI 95%
Hyperstimulation syndrome	n. e.		
Uterine dehiscence / rupture	n. e.		
Genital or perineal trauma	8'102	8 (0.1)	0.1 - 0.2
Mild or moderate vaginal bleeding	3'816	23 (0.6)	0.4 - 0.9
Heavy vaginal bleeding	7'037	1'837 (26.1)	25.1 - 27.1
Other intrapartum complications	12'573	82 (0.7)	0.5 - 0.8
Caesarean section	n. e.		
Total	n. e.		

Birth outcome: Sublingual application

	Cervical ripening and labour induction		
	N women	ADR (%)	CI 95 %
Event			
Uterine contraction abnormalities without FHRch	443	61 (13.8)	10.9 - 17.3
Hyperstimulation syndrome	568	37 (6.5)	4.8 - 8.8
Uterine dehiscence/rupture	n. e.		
Genital or perineal trauma	n. e.		
Mild or moderate vaginal bleeding	899	355 (39.5)	36.3 - 42.7
Heavy vaginal bleeding	756	4 (0.5)	0.2 - 1.4
Caesarean section	568	150 (26.4)	23.0 - 30.2

Abortion induction and prevention of PPH were not evaluated for outcome of birth.

Neonatal ADR: Sublingual application

	N newborns	ADR (%)	CI 95%
ADR			
Apgar score ≤6 at 5 min	568	14 (2.5)	1.5 - 4.1
Admission to NICU	568	44 (7.7)	5.8 - 10.2
Presence of signs of foetal distress	568	275 (48.4)	44.3 - 52.5
Neonatal death	n. e.		
Other neonatal ADR	n.e.		

More Books!

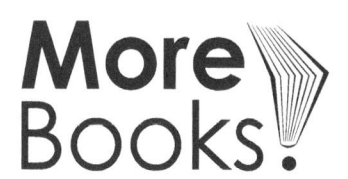

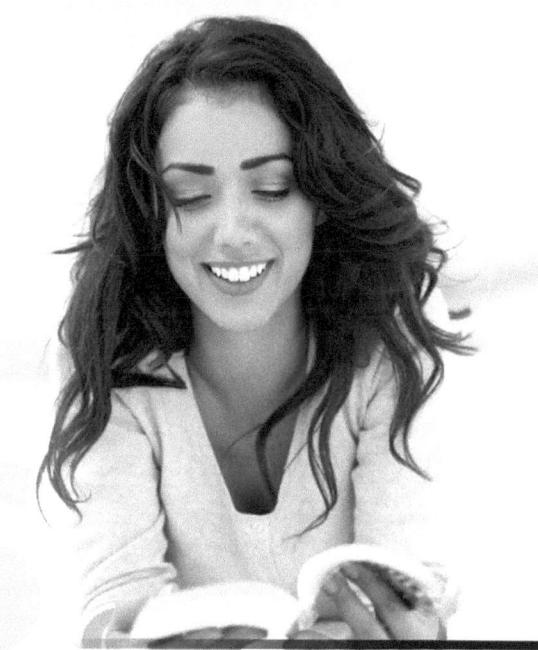

i want morebooks!

Buy your books fast and straightforward online - at one of world's fastest growing online book stores! Environmentally sound due to Print-on-Demand technologies.

Buy your books online at
www.get-morebooks.com

Kaufen Sie Ihre Bücher schnell und unkompliziert online – auf einer der am schnellsten wachsenden Buchhandelsplattformen weltweit! Dank Print-On-Demand umwelt- und ressourcenschonend produziert.

Bücher schneller online kaufen
www.morebooks.de

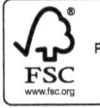

Printed by Books on Demand GmbH, Norderstedt / Germany